Exposing her vulnerability and show-casing her strength … this wonderful book of poetry … lly demonstrates that, while she … n.

… or

Every now and then a poetry … another place. One minute you … the next hot lava is slowly poured on you from a height. Samantha can arouse feelings that appeared dead or dormant for years. A stunning piece of work.

Paul Cooper, actor, writer and hoarding disorder advocate

I have long believed in the therapeutic power of poetry as someone who turned to words that heal during my own depressive episodes. Samantha Crilly is an accomplished poet whose own inspirational writing about her mental illness powerfully illuminates what it is to suffer. But Crilly's work is also about fostering strength and giving us words for recovery. Her new book is a 'must-read' for anyone looking for literary solace and companionship as the darkness recedes and resilience returns.

Rachel Kelly, *Sunday Times* bestselling author of *Black Rainbow: How words healed me – my journey through depression*

A beautiful soul leaps off the page full of hope, vulnerability and a breath-taking self-awareness. I could read these poems again and again each time feeling something new.

Mikyla Dodd, actress, writer and counsellor

To my twin sister Charlotte

My first friend, lifelong confidante and mirror soul –
Thank you for sharing every heartbeat of this
journey with me,
Your strength, laughter and love have
shaped me more than words can say.
This book is as much yours as it is mine.

SAMANTHA CRILLY

Strength Through Poetry

Resilience in rhythm:
The strength of mind and body in verse

With a Foreword by Frank Bruno MBE
With illustrations by Sarah Lou

HH BOOKS

Hammersmith Health Books
London, UK

First published in 2026 by Hammersmith Health Books
– an imprint of Hammersmith Books Limited
82 Wandsworth Bridge Road, London, SW6 2TF
www.hammersmithbooks.co.uk

British Library Cataloguing in Publication Data:
A CIP record of this book is available from the British Library.

Print ISBN 978-1-78161-286-6
Ebook ISBN 978-1-78161-287-3

Commissioning editor: Georgina Bentliff
Illustrations: Sarah Lou
Designed and typeset by: Madeline Meckiffe
Cover design by: Madeline Meckiffe
Cover illustrations: Shutterstock/Tartila
Index: Hammersmith Books Limited
Production: Anke Ueberberg
Printed and bound by: T J Books, UK

MIX
Paper | Supporting responsible forestry
FSC® C013056
www.fsc.org

Contents

Foreword by Frank Bruno MBE 9
My story 11

Poems about family and relationships 13

Two souls, one heart – a poem dedicated to my twin sister Charlotte 15
Hands that build – a poem dedicated to my dad 16
A wise old owl – a poem dedicated to my grandma 19
The heart that held me – a poem about my mother's love 20
Paws in heaven – a poem about losing a pet dog 22

Poems about states of mind 23

When the shadows speak back – a poem about sitting with your own thoughts 24
Away with the fairies – a poem about daydreaming with the devil 26
Endless circles – a poem about over-thinking 28
Lake of hearts – a poem about heartbreak 31
The devil's flowers – a poem about – living with disordered eating 32
Surviving the Sun – a poem about making it through the day. .33
The quiet face of night – a poem about good days and bad days 35
Echoes after good-bye – a poem about grief 36
The grace of silver years – a poem about ageing 37

Poems about mental health challenges 39

Knock knock – a poem about addiction 40
You and I – a poem about bipolar 41
Handcuffed – a poem about mental illness 42
Between bite and breath – a poem about anorexia nervosa ... 44
Not my face – a poem about gender dysphoria 45
Between walls and wires – a poem about hoarding disorder from a carer's perspective 47
Fight or flight – a poem about PTSD 48
One bite – a poem about the distorted relationship with food 50
The silence between words – a poem about dementia 53
Pills and promises – a poem about medication 54
Tangled currents – a poem about ADHD 55
The beast – a poem about the beast that is mental illness 56
The loop I live in – a poem about OCD 58
The purge – a poem about bulimia 59
When the walls cave in – a poem about anxiety 60

Poems about the challenges of contemporary life 63

Doom scroll – a poem about the dark side of social media ... 64
Hell under heaven – a poem about masking how you feel 65
Girl of the trees – a poem about being different 66
Hollow hours – a poem about loneliness 69
Models of diversity – a poem about diversity in the fashion industry 70
I am man – a poem about the unspoken struggles that men experience 72
Scroll and hollow – a poem about social media 74
Roots – a poem about our environment 76
The troll – a poem about cyber bullying 78
Rhyme – a poem about the effects of modern life 79

Poems about the emotional challenges of physical health issues 81

My cage – a poem about Parkinson's disease 82
A broken house – a poem about multiple sclerosis 83
Eyes of the soul – a poem about blindness 85
The heat of change – a poem about menopause 86
The music I imagine – a poem about deafness 88
The quiet ache – a poem about arthritis 89
Threads of hope – a poem about cancer 91
The weight of waking – a poem about chronic fatigue syndrome 92

Poems about positivity 95

Steady in the storm – a poem from a carer to a sufferer 96
Hands that heal – a poem about being kind 97
My gift – a poem about loving your body 99
I shall not judge – a poem about not judging people 100
The heart I hold – a poem about self-love 101
My lighthouse – from a sufferer to a carer 102
Outside the ring – a poem dedicated to Frank Bruno 105
Where the stars whisper hope – a poem about hope 108
We all bleed the same – a poem about communities coming together 110
Malcolm 111

Resources and support 112
Acknowledgements 118
Index 119

Foreword

By Frank Bruno MBE

I was never all that good at school. I didn't listen. I was more interested in getting home and getting down to the boxing gym. That's probably why I ended up being sent to a 'special school' for naughty kids. Well, that's what they called it. Truth was, it was a borstal. Either way, it certainly straightened me out!

Looking back, I wish I'd listened a bit more in English classes. I'd love to be a bit better with my writing and spelling. Why? Well one thing I've found in my life is words can be just as powerful as your fists. The little pep-talks I had between rounds from my trainer, George Francis, God rest his soul, will always live long in the memory. 'One more round, Frank,' George famously said to me before the 12th round of my fight with Oliver McCall, 'Three minutes 'till you're a Champ. Three minutes till we're at the top of the mountain.'

Words helped me too when I hit rock bottom. When I was lying in a hospital bed in a psychiatric ward after being sectioned, I'd read the Serenity Prayer over and over again. It gave me hope. It helped me to fight. It helped me come back.

So, yeah, I know better than anyone that words can be really powerful.

And that's why I'm so proud to write this Foreword for this amazing new book by Samantha Crilly. I've known Samantha for a few years now. When she first sent me some of her poetry, I was blown away by it. She even wrote one about my life which was so amazing I turned it into a video and now play it at the start of the shows which I take around the country. People who attend often stop and ask me at the end about the poem* and say how much they enjoyed it.

Samantha's a fighter. She's had challenges. But thanks to her resilience, and the love and support of her friends and family, especially her mum Lynn, dad Kevin and twin-sister Charlotte, she's winning that battle. But even more importantly she's using her own experiences to now try and help others.

Since retiring I've tried to do that too. I've tried to offer others a little bit of hope when all they can see is despair. I've tried to offer a bit of light at the end of the tunnel. Samantha's amazing poems do all of that and more. Which is why I am super-grateful that Sam and her family have agreed to give some of the proceeds of her book to my own charity, the Frank Bruno Foundation. This gesture means Samantha's words will now help many others fighting their own battles.

God Bless,
Frank Bruno MBE
Former Heavyweight Boxing World Champion, founder of The Frank Bruno Mental Health Foundation and author of *60 Years A Fighter*. To buy a copy visit: www.frankbruno.co.uk/shop

* This poem is on page 105

My story

Thank you for taking the time to look at this book and to read my poetry. I hope that you will take a positive message from my writing, recognising that a glimmer and shimmer of light can be found even through dark and challenging times.

Writing this book has been a cathartic experience for me, helping me find a way to express thoughts and words that can often be hard to say out loud. Committing my feelings to paper calms me, helps me unravel difficult emotions, and shows me just how far I have come. I hope reading my verses will help you in a similar way. You will also find pages dedicated to your own thoughts and ideas here and there throughout the book so you too can find ways of committing challenging emotions to paper.

Writing poetry has been a helpful, healthy and positive way of organising the sea of emotions I have often felt adrift in. Over the years I have expressed these feeling through far more destructive paths. From the age of 13, I spiralled into the grip of an eating disorder which put a huge strain on both me and my family throughout my teenage years. Then, as I felt that recovery was almost within my reach, I swapped one mental illness for another, becoming ill with obsessive compulsive disorder. Once again, the order I sought eluded me, and my life felt very out of control.

Finally in my mid-20s, with the unwavering support of my family and friends, I found three great passions – drama, script writing and poetry – all giving me a creative outlet and a home for my imagination which has been crucial to my recovery. I achieved a degree in stage and media, and as I became happier and more self- confident, I found myself much more committed to writing. I can now look back and see that, as each poem takes its shape and form, I moved a little further forward towards long-lasting health and happiness.

To be here now, as the author of my second poetry book, feels quite surreal and exciting. I hope that all who read it will find strength and understanding through its pages. I am not an academic, nor a trained writer; I am simply a young woman writing from the heart about real things that matter to me, and some have said that is the most powerful thing about my poetry.

Over the last year I have enjoyed writing these poems so much and I hope that comes across to those who read them. I hope they will show that if you believe in yourself, your capabilities and dreams, then you can move forward in a strong, healthy and hopeful way. Those steps you take may be tiny, but they add up over time and now, in a much healthier place, I can see how far I have come. Sometimes I feel frustration that there is still a little way to go, but if I have learnt anything, it is that this journey cannot be rushed.

I am so incredibly grateful to all those who have encouraged me to get here and have let me follow my own path at my own pace, which has led to this book that you are holding in your hands today. Twenty years ago, in the grip of anorexia nervosa, I hardly dared to think about the future. From that dark, frightening place I could never have imagined the sunshine that I would be standing in now.

Poems about family and relationships

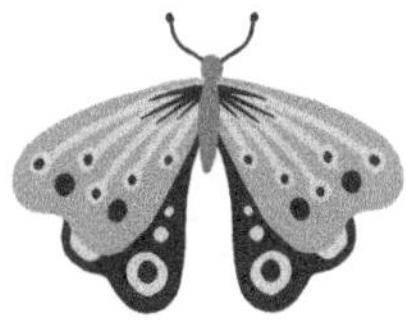

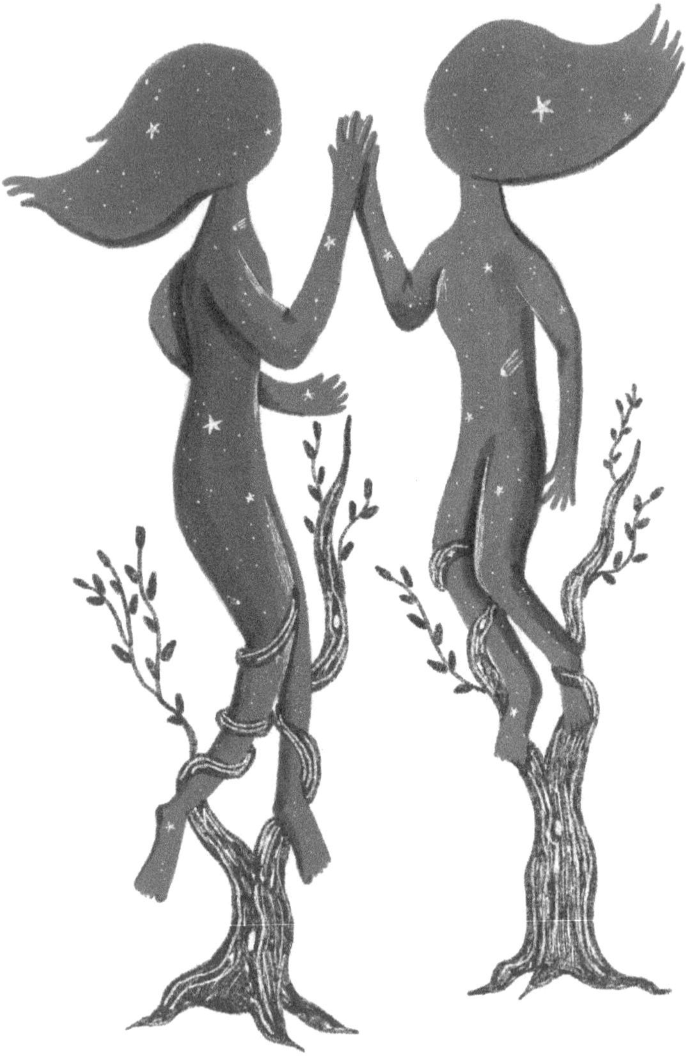

Two souls, one heart

A poem dedicated to my twin sister Charlotte

It's our history that's draped upon us in robes
Our souls sheltered by shoes from the same wardrobe
A reminder upon the face of each
That even through squalls, a love can cease to impeach
That you are in me and I am in you
Our past, present and future will always be one yet two
A companion I never earned yet was gifted
For my wings to work, to keep them lifted
You are the beauty that floods in through pain
My life's soulmate again and again

Hands that build

A poem dedicated to my dad

It's a strength that needs no words
Like the wind beneath the birds.
It quietly carries you through
moments of falling apart.
He'll subtly arrive with the glue,
Nothing deep said beyond the ocean floor,
But he'll build a boat to take you safely to shore.
A love that sits in your shadow through good and pain
Pull a tissue out of his pocket with no need to explain.

My thoughts

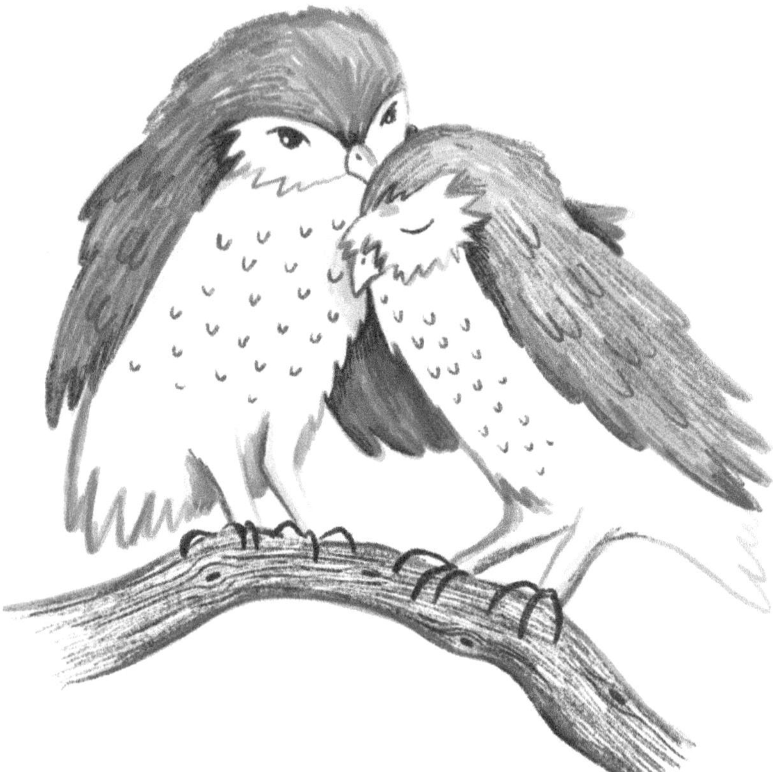

A wise old owl

A poem dedicated to my grandma

A wise old owl has always been near
To whisper words of wisdom in my ear
Life years I haven't yet lived or learned
The lessons where knowledge can only be earned
Oh, to have such a place to go with queries of concern
A loving perspective but also firm
You, my grandma, have been my bird in the trees
Sending all my answers through the ever-moving breeze
One day I'll be wise, I'll know what to do
But in the meantime, I'll come and sit next to you

The heart that held me

A poem about my mother's love

You're my best friend whom I adore
You taught me everything I know
and more
You never abandoned me
when times got tough
You held my trembling hands
when things got rough
You have always been by my side.
Holding me up when I wanted to hide
The friendship we have is so rare to find
For a mother and daughter to have combined
We have been there for each other when
we have laughed and cried
We feel each other's pain if we hurt inside
The miles between us can't tear us apart
Because we will keep each other close in our hearts

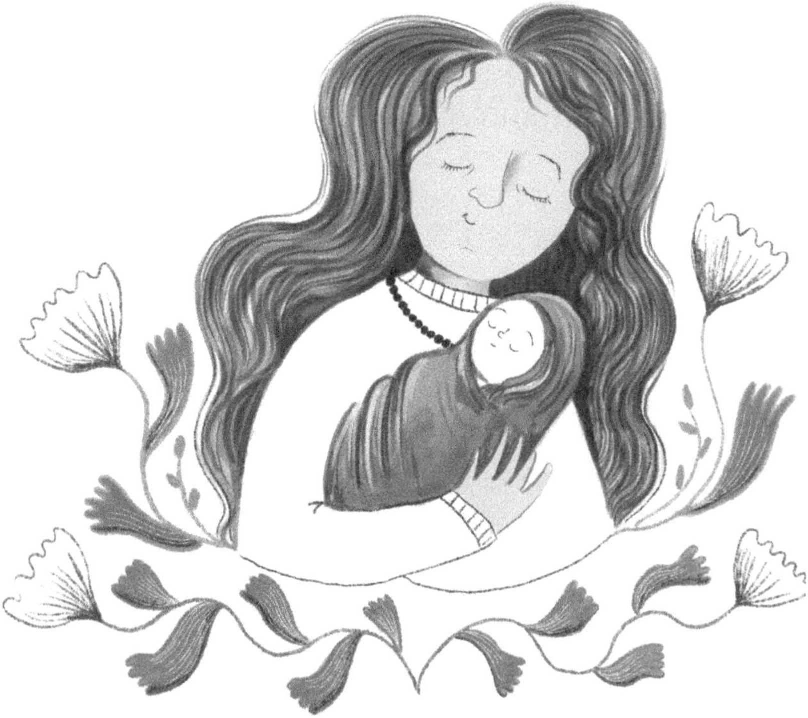

Paws in heaven

A poem about losing a pet dog

Up in heaven my paws pull the clouds.
As I look down on my old muddy grounds
I see you still walk the route we would share.
It still looks just as beautiful even though I am not there.
I hope when you walk you look up to the sun,
As that's me up there running about having fun.
When you get to our favourite view
The breeze you feel on your skin is me next to you.
I'm still here, though in spirit as they say,
I still love to watch your routines of the day.
I miss you and everyone else too,
But I know they will hold your heart and help you through.
And when you arrive home at 6 pm,
At least you'll now know your slippers are where you left them.
Sometimes in the night's hours I see you cry for me,
But I had to find peace up here in this world pain free.
One day we will walk again on the same misty turf,
Our love will always override the distance
between heaven and earth.

Poems about states of mind

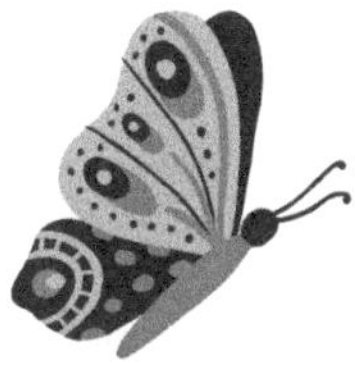

When the shadows speak back

A poem about sitting with your own thoughts

When I'm done laughing, smiling away,
When I've cracked my last joke, when I'm done with the day,
I'll sit in my room quietly tucked away
from the mask on my face
to make it look like I'm okay.
To some it's a peaceful time with no act to follow,
For others it's a darker moment with no happy pill to swallow.
There are nights the quiet helps to reset my head;
Others I lie side by side conversing with the demons on my bed.

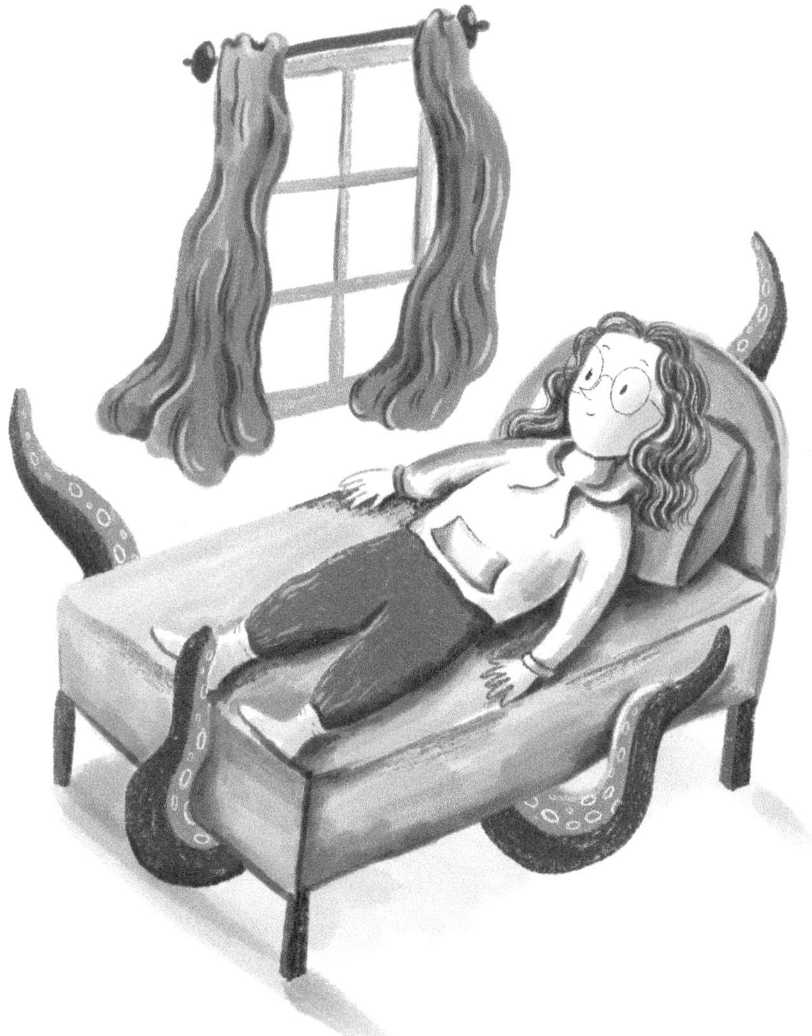

Away with the fairies

A poem about daydreaming with the devil

People always say I am away with the fairies,
singing along, picking berries.
Oh, how I wish such magic would surround me.
Instead, I'm conversing with the monster that found me.
Such enhancement does't exist; if only I could say
That it's the devil not the angels taking me away.

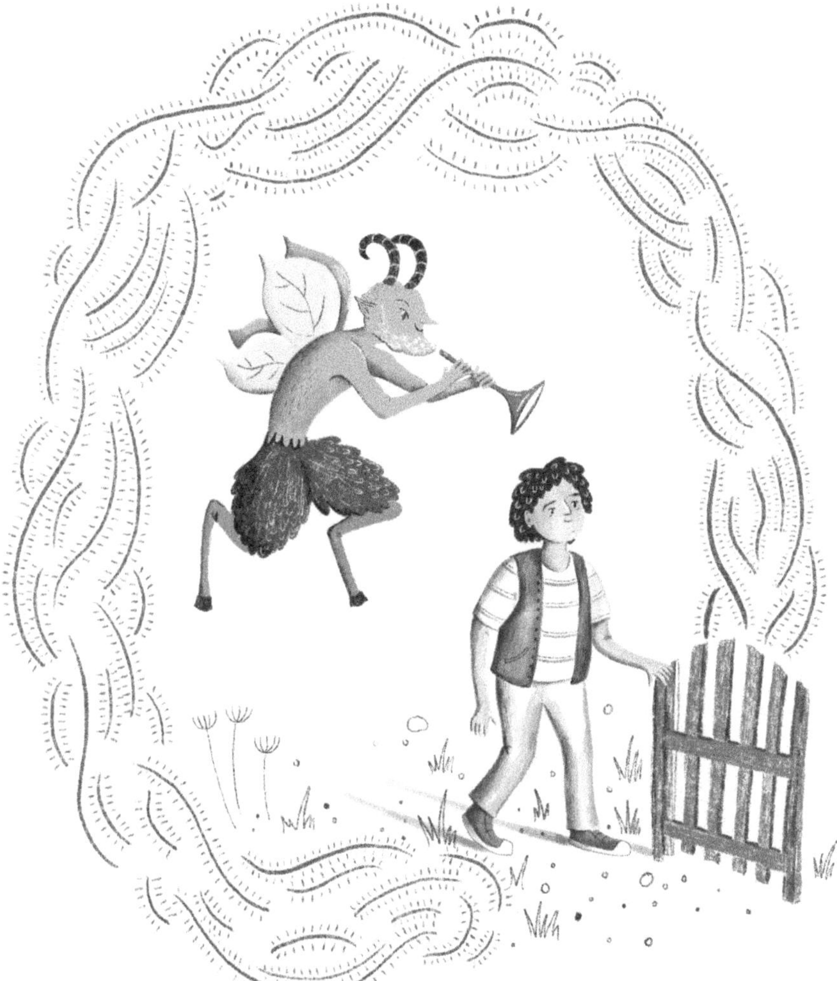

Endless circles

A poem about over-thinking

It's the silence that always gets me
Within that sudden moment of clarity
As I drive home alone
no music, no voices, a quiet phone
Often leaves me breathless in my own convictions
Self-sabotaging with no optimistic prescriptions
Was I too much? Was I too less?
Did I lay bare more than one should confess?
Truth is, I don't know, well probably not
Most likely they're worrying about dinner or putting the baby to sleep in its cot
My tongue for them will soon be just a feeble memory
Whereas for me it's always an instant regrettable enemy
So, I'll try not to think too much about what has gone wrong
For there will be another scenario I'll over-think before too long

My thoughts

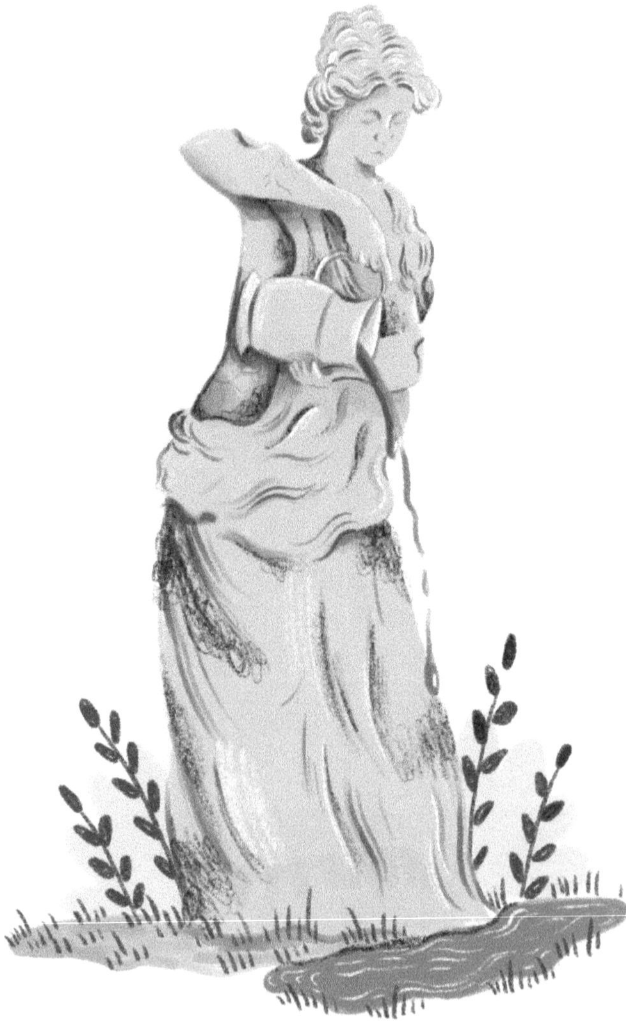

Lake of hearts

A poem
about heartbreak

My heart will sliver down winding roads
Fall into murky waters and kiss a few toads
Be enticed into dark forests by a slight glimmer on a leaf
Only to be stolen by a night crawling thief
Who will grip it for a while as it cracks in their hands
A once strong sculpture can soon vanish to sand
But I will always receive it back as I pick up each piece
Every part will still be there for me to fill in each crease
Whole again, although not as smooth as once was
I know it can take a punch which always deserves applause
In moments like these you will feel like you're alone,
lost in life's game
Left in a lake of what seems like everlasting pain
But little do you know it will be brimming
with hearts just the same
Perhaps you will connect, or perhaps you won't
But one thing you will realise is that you were never alone

The devil's flowers

A poem about living with disordered eating

Hello, as the author, I am here
in the wind, in the rain to speak kind words in your ear
I know you lie awake through the night's hours
For food has now shifted into the devil's flowers
It inhabits your mind – that you should be punished
When its true mantra is just to coexist
Let it play as your antidote, a nourishing role
Not for punishment as a means of control
An addiction it seems has you under its thumb
But it was not put here for you to gorge, then after feel numb
Or to be counted in numbers, revised in excess
To give you no pleasure, only to summon stress
I know these illnesses have you on puppet strings
That they've crawled right under all your skins
Know you are worthy of being free, you are worth so much more
Than all these rules which have brought your knees to the floor
I believe in you, so fiercely with all my heart
Don't let these disorders tear you apart

Surviving the sun

A poem about making it through the day

Most people dread the dark nights,
Roads lined with glaring streetlights.
As the Sun sets eagerly over the winter months,
My goodness, I used to begrudge it too once.
Now, the earlier I can see an end to the day
I find myself celebrating in a small way.
As I breathe a sigh of relief that I made it through
Even though there is no glorious Sun in my view.
I know the day is done, I made it out okay.
My demons were successfully kept at bay.
Oh, how I would love to have the want for more time,
More hours in the day to hold as mine.
However, I know one day I'll look up at the sky.
My feet nestled in the grass as the Sun passes by,
And I'll never want it to leave; I'll cherish its stay,
As my demons will at that point be somewhere far away.

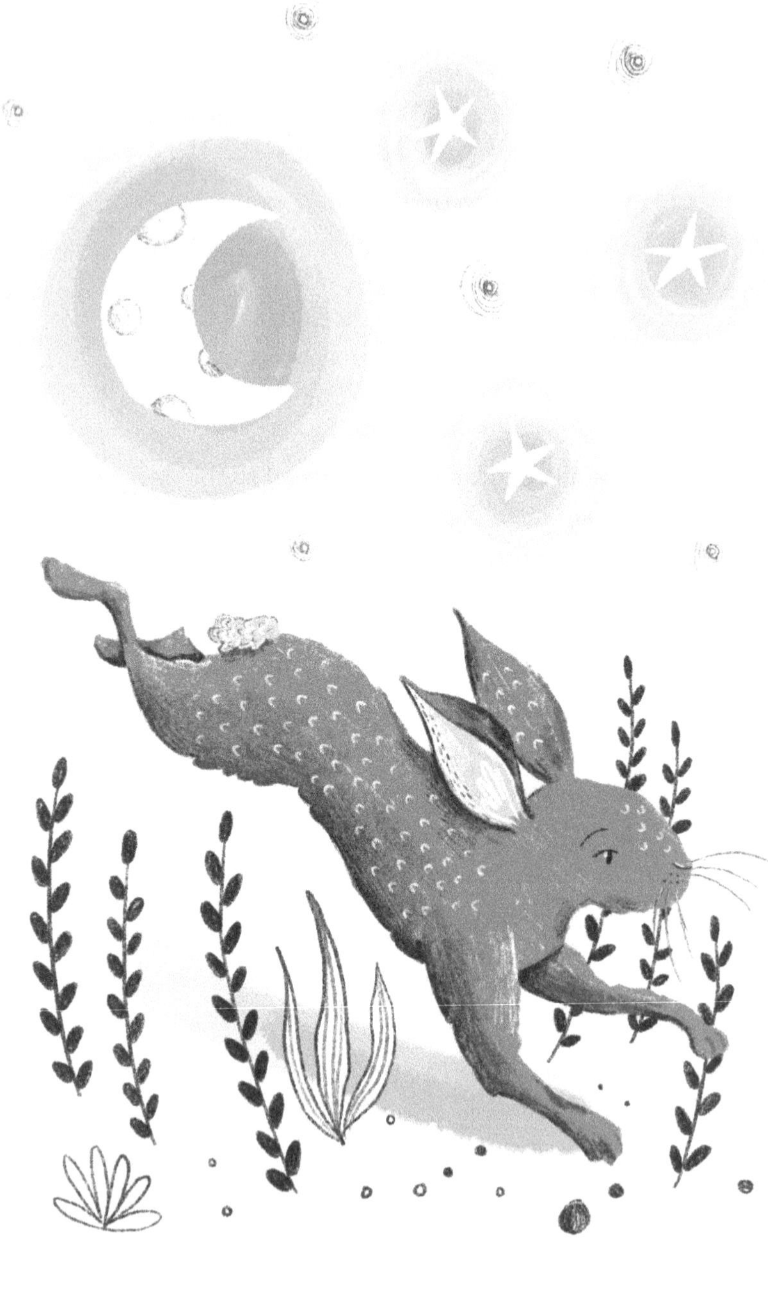

The quiet face of night

A poem about good days and bad days

When the moon shines upon me at night
Although on scattered evenings it may not be bright
For then it only half shows its face
The rest will always sit up in space.
This is me at times I now know.
My whole light will not always show
But it will be waiting, in anticipation, to reappear
On the darker days I now cease to fear.

Echoes after goodbye

A poem about grief

They took my heart with them when they passed
The love you have for your child never surrenders fast
It's like an ocean; it comes in waves, receding and flowing
Like the wind, it never stops blowing
Sometimes the water is subtle, sometimes it spins
All you can do is learn to swim.

The grace of silver years

A poem about ageing

And in the end do we ever find solace until we are old and grey?
Only when we find ourselves with much less time to waste away
Do we sit peacefully within the comfort of our own minds
Without a quorum of who's peeking through our blinds
Passing judgement on everything we do
Because let's be honest there are only very few
And the faults we once thought our body held
Are beautiful things that took us through this world.
If only such peace that time can bring
Would come earlier and calm the worrying.

My thoughts

Poems about mental health challenges

Knock knock

A poem about addiction

A knock at the door, I answered with glee,
A handsome stranger staring back at me.
Take my arm, I'll give you all the answers, they said.
I was soon in love after a lustful night in bed.
They became my antidote, I was addicted,
Life seemed finer than I could ever have predicted.
This was it, until they soon changed
into some kind of demon, unhinged and deranged.
Oh, believe me I tried so many times to leave
But they always had a clever trick up their sleeve.
To think we had such a bright future planned,
For them to only tear me apart then lend me their hand.
Many people go to them with the hope of making it through to the other side
Only when it's all gone, is it revealed that they have lied.
Your answers will always rest within that one person
Who you already knew –
That person will always and only ever be you.

You and I

A poem about bipolar

We run alongside each other, you and I
My other entity from the sky.
You often come down when I'm on a high
Only to dampen and drop a tear in my eye.
You spill your case of thoughts, ready for me to unpack
Then run away before I have time to give it all back.
I'll lie there in the night as the moon sits high
Trying my very best not to lie there and cry.
You'll visit again like a beam of light,
Retrieve me from the depths, everything will seem bright.
I will dance in this haven till I see you anew
Before the next suitcase I know will be due.

Handcuffed

A poem about mental illness

Imagine if cancer was a person.
How they would look, what they would say,
How they would manipulate you in every single way,
The evil which would seep through their eyes,
Their foul words and repellent lies.
The crown they'd gladly place upon their head,
To indoctrinate you with every word they have said.
A scent you would so dreadfully smell
From their breath of life being spent unwell.
A face gaunt, hanging in the wind,
Hair greasy as oil, body worn and thinned.
Now imagine being handcuffed to them 24/7.
My god, you could only pray it gets better in heaven.
This is how one who suffers with a mental illness lives,
Side by side with an entity that never gives.
Be kind, allow them time to rest,
For the next day they can again only try their very best.

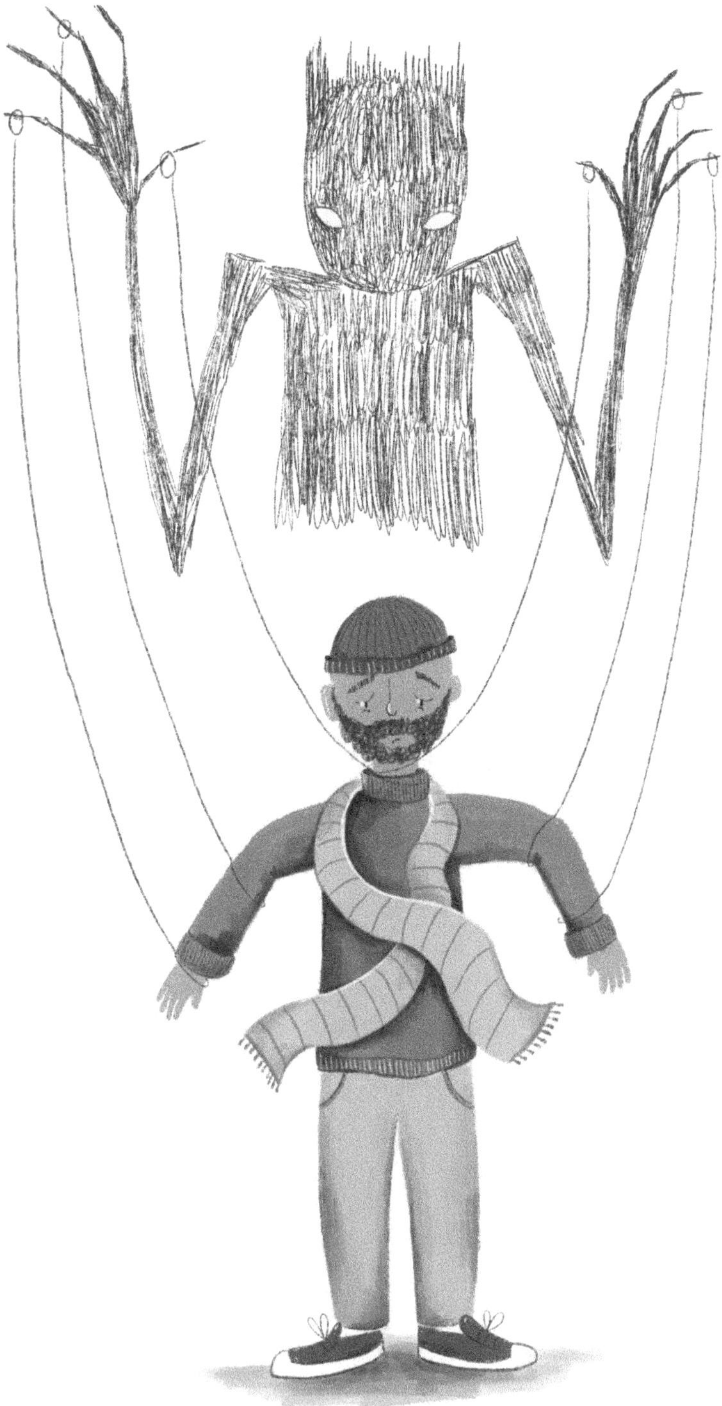

Between bite and breath

A poem about anorexia nervosa

It was a friendly hand taking me into a dark space
A smile of glee painted upon her face
It appeared enchanting, a place I'd never been
I could become a version of myself no one had ever seen
Ana, she called herself, so soft and so subtle
Little did I know her words meant only trouble
She was 'it', she was my leader, my ruler, my feeder
To my body, to my mind, but my goodness did she become unkind
She feasted on my bones, my weakness for control
She knew she could play with an impressionable soul
For that she is a devil in angel's wear
Compelling me to survive only on fresh air
But demons can only wear fancy dress for so long without show
For the seeds soon die when you have rotten ones to sow
So, when you think back on her in your mind
Make sure you remember the wicked and unkind
Because that is all you have truly left behind

Not my face

A poem about gender dysphoria

In the mirror a stranger's face
Reflections twist in a silent space
Clothes that fit like a cage so tight
Dreams of freedom in the dead of night
Voices whisper you don't belong
Yet deep inside the truth is strong
The body feels like a borrowed shell
Somewhere I live but don't know well
I will one day wear clothes that allow me to breathe
In the light air as I roll up my sleeves
I look in the mirror at my own face
That carries my soul in its suitcase
If I'm patient, I know I will see
A place of freedom through finding me

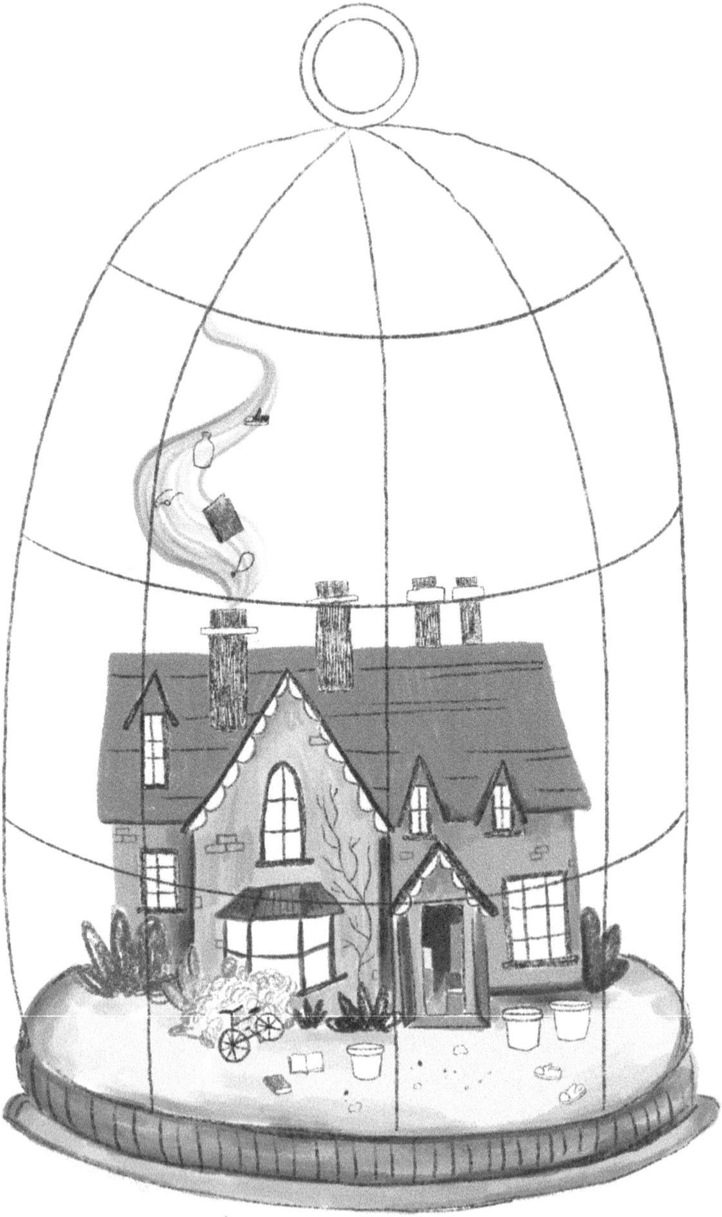

Between walls and wires

A poem about hoarding disorder from a carer's perspective

There are pretty things
and useful things of no use
Broken cables, dusty birthday banners
My old childhood shoes
Drenched upon entering, I step on 1990s news
Do you still see me with a house so full and unclean,
With piles of paper in between us; I know I can't be seen
I often wonder if you still want me here
As the magazines being gone not me is really your biggest fear
I know memories lie deep within them
Even secrets you haven't shared
Memorials of friends and family for grief you haven't aired
Moving into the future has you mighty scared
My dearest mother, you now sit alone
For a once soulful house, now has no one home
Apart from ghosts who walk the corners
Our old selves still take a stroll
As you wither to your knees alone, restrained by its control

Fight or flight

A poem about PTSD

It never leaves you, the fight.
The smell, the taste, the deep rooted blight,
Now growing upon my days, winding its way through
any peace and solace that I once knew.
Hounded by my regiment as if I'm still on duty.
Letting the world just flow, still seems so new to me.
I latch onto the control, who could suffer if I lose?
Who will be hindered by each bad decision I choose?
Anxiety, paranoia, ripple through each vein.
For every bloodshed I witnessed I constantly feel the pain.
But every day I fight through is a success as far as I'm concerned.
Something that over time I have come to have learned.
I will never stop fighting, even if it's in my head.
The silent battle I will now win instead.

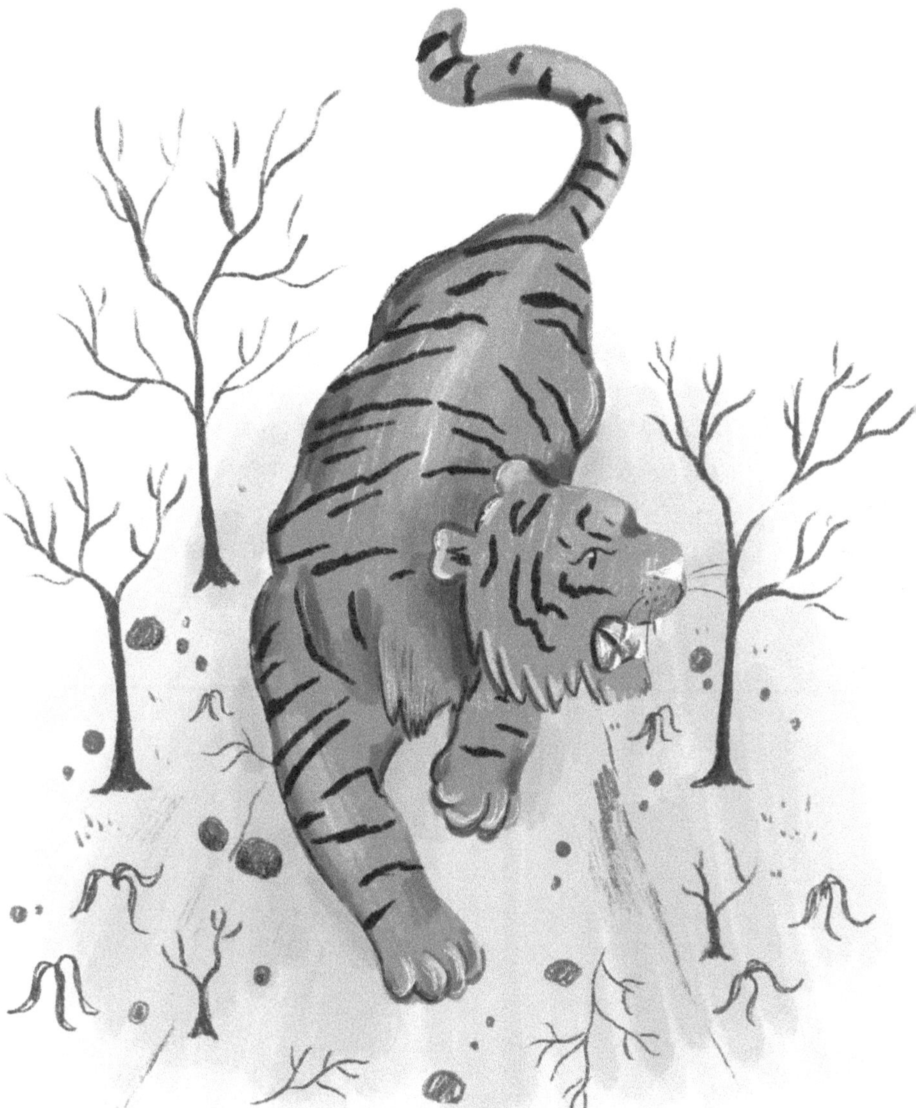

One bite

A poem about the distorted relationship with food

I hope the dust settles one day.
Life would be much more peaceful that way.
As we live alongside each other, you and me,
Your whisper I hear in my ear constantly,
On whether that bite will be really worth it
Or if you will then taunt me for not being perfect?
Sure, I know all the right things to do,
But perhaps sometimes you'll let me feed my soul too?
To not agonise so much about the guilty discussion,
To cherish each bite without any repercussion.
No more calories or labels to scan and fine tune,
Just to choose with lust, can we get there soon?
As I'm so ready to live for myself and be free
Without rules, without guilt and an apology.

My thoughts

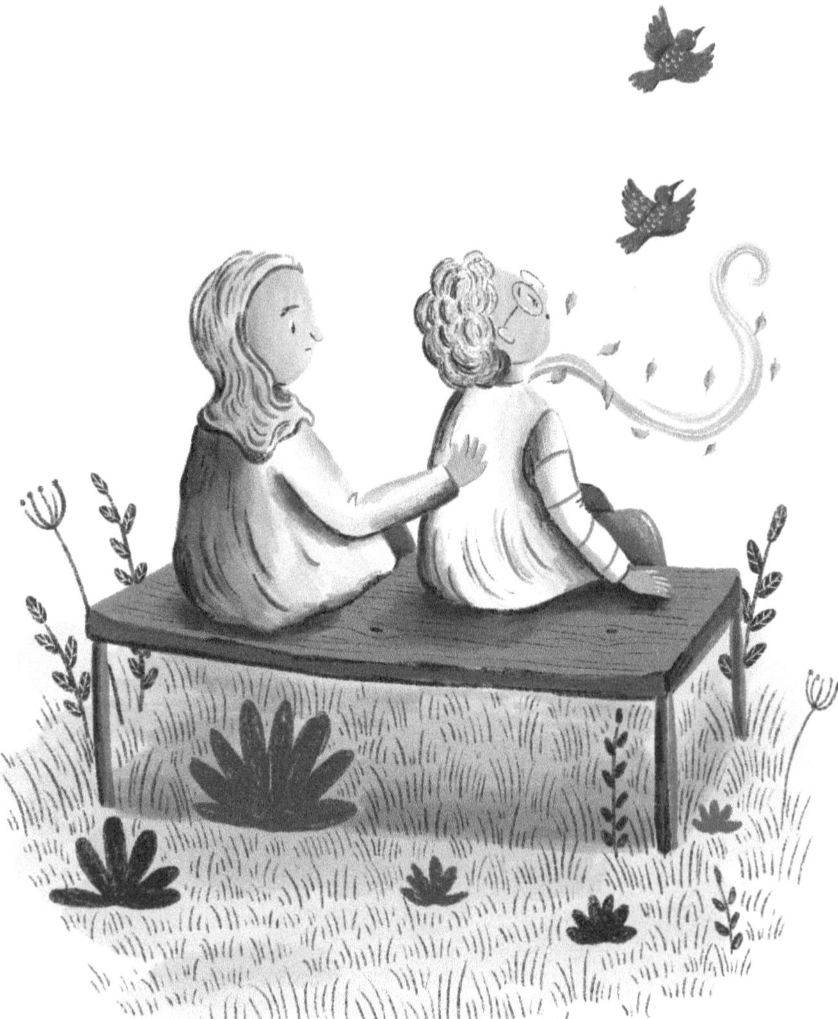

The silence between words

A poem about dementia

Some people ask why I still come
Why would I subject myself to something so numb?
Why do I still talk to you with no replies?
Why I still stare into your desolate eyes
without any feeling of upset?
Truth is, I do, I just know it's not over yet
There is still that odd moment, I catch that glint in your eye,
You say my name for a second, and then say goodbye
But just that second of you makes it all worthwhile,
To have you look back at me with your beautiful smile.
Say my name like you have since the day of my birth
Oh, I will do this every day until your body leaves this earth.
Even if your soul reaches heaven beyond
Every little piece of you here I will always hold on.

Pills and promises

A poem about medication

It's chaos living here, within my mind.
I would scrape the barrel, desperate for any peace I can find.
I always doubted medication, worried it would change
my wires too much.
That I would lose my essence, my own touch.
But when in mayhem, you will try anything
to get yourself out of this relentless ring.
The chaos did subside, even though it's still inside.
Thankfully it is quieter, as it lies at the back,
In the shadows of my mind. I like that.
I may be a little slower, sometimes more weary,
The side effects aren't always the most cheery,
But it has never changed who I am. I am still me.
I am still myself, just a little more free.

Tangled currents

A poem about ADHD

My mind holds stars, too fast to trace,
They shoot so quick, they won't stay in place.
My thoughts bloom like wildflowers do,
In colours no one ever drew.
Where others walk, I sometimes fly—
Not on the ground, but through the sky.
But where others drown I can often swim.
I can see bright light when the lamps are dim.
Though my storms may seem like flaws,
It's a power used to open unworking doors.
So don't mistake my scattered ways
For something broken, far away.
There's magic in the ever-moving sea
For I am it and it is me.

The beast

A poem about the beast that is mental illness

You know those moments you crave alone,
When people have worn you down to the bone,
As you sit in your car watching the sun go down
Or soak in a warm bath with no one else around.
These are the moments that keep us sane,
The ones we need again and again,
Allowing us to un-muddle the chaos in our mind,
To leave the hectic day behind.
Oh, how I wish I could feel such peace.
As always, perched next to me sits the wicked beast.
It strikes me with its infectious warts,
Whilst feasting lavishly on all my thoughts.
It's no wonder I have lost my mind,
As its pallet of words is always brimming with bile,
Telling me I have no motive in my existence to smile,
To be joyous of life, so if it seems I can struggle.
Please understand I am not weak but strong.
To stay and survive this beast for so long.

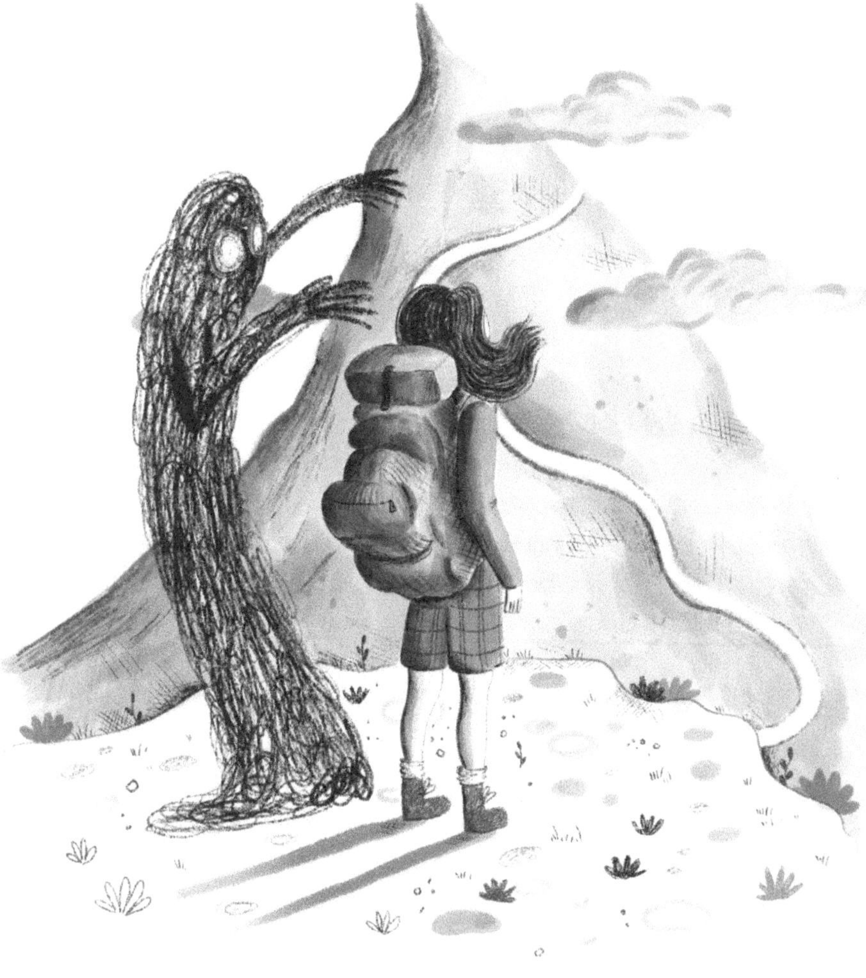

The loop I live in

A poem about OCD

Whispers in my mind unravel me like lace,
'Do it once more, just in case.'
The switch is turned, again, once more,
Though it clicked ten times — I am never sure.
The stove is cold, the iron's still,
But my palm still lurches to have one last feel.
Hands scrubbed profusely with soap till raw,
Lines of blood flake my knuckles as they lie sore.
Shoes aligned, a spotless floor,
I shan't stop; there is always more.
Tilted pictures and pillows I align each day
Even if it takes the morning sunrise away.
I know it lies, but will always plead,
Yet still it bends me to my knee.
It borrows logic; from a mad man it buys
Rules which are wrapped in lies.
All the loops and rituals that fill my head
Dismantle my sleep as I lie in bed.
Stay strong as the mad man will always be mad.
He will always sit lurking in the shadows making me feel bad.
So, please remember, on days his power feels tall,
That inside his might will always be small.

The purge

A poem about bulimia

In quiet rooms and empty streets
I find a place to start my feast—
A banquet built from borrowed peace,
As I fill my hands for a quick release.
The heights can reach that of cocaine
Leading me without any restraint.
Bent in prayer, I spill my sin
Trying to erase the war within.
I'll discard as soon as the high retrieves,
Open the toilet lid, pull up my sleeves.
It slices through the skin in my throat
As the devil holds my ego, and starts to stroke.
It'll laugh at me, all proud and smug
As I sit on my knees, its victim, a mug.
I'll stand on my feet and prevail through
As an angel calls, 'This is not what to do.
You are more than calories, you're more than food,
You're more than this wine the devil has brewed.'
I follow my angel in times of need,
In times when I can start to feel a feed
There's light; there's hope;
There are so many better ways to cope.

When the walls cave in

A poem about anxiety

It lingers like a second skin
Never knowing when it will seep it.
I feel its hands, nestle up my spine
As the monster starts to grab a hold of my mind.
It climbs and clutches every inch of my chest
As it pulls like a corset till nothing is left.
Past, present and future co-exist in one
As time stops and my brain becomes numb.
Is this panic or have I touched death?
Is this what it feels like when no time is left?
People smudged like watercolour dripping,
Voices blend in the midst of my own ripping,
But still – breath returns, shallow at first,
A fragile truce to delay my hearse
And slowly the world rebuilds its shape
From the invisible reality of my own earthquake.

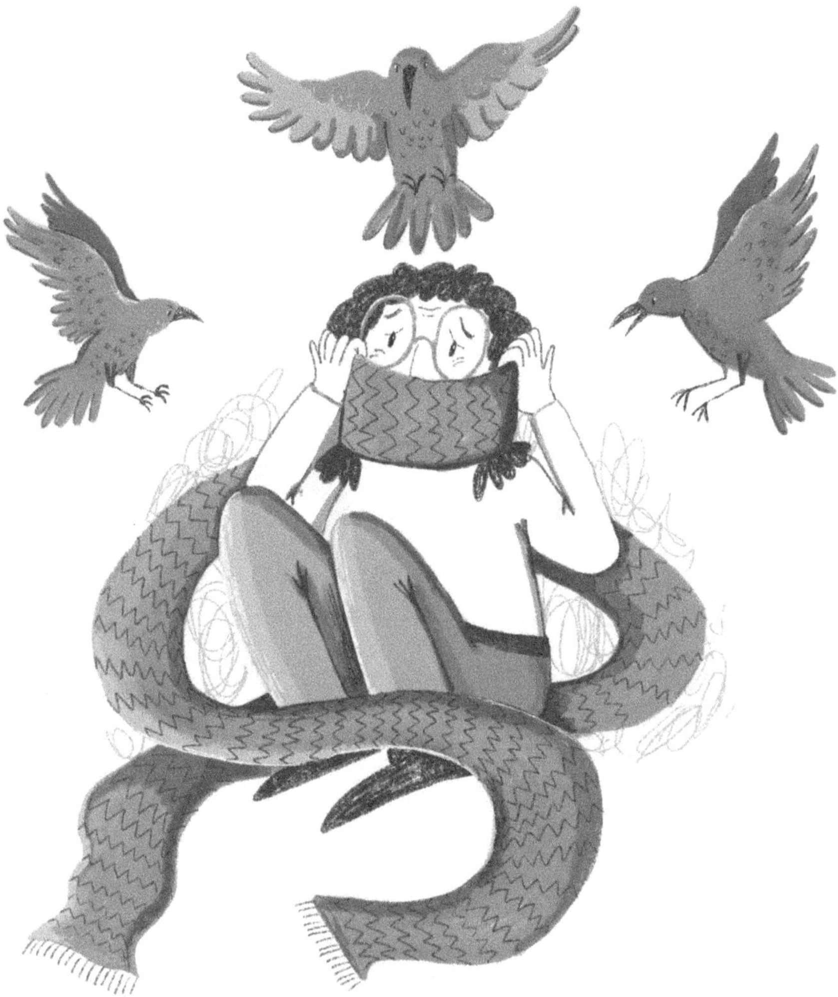

My thoughts

Poems about the challenges of contemporary life

Doom scroll

A poem about the dark side of social media

I'll sit in the midst of the night,
At lunch in between each bite,
In the morning, the first thing I do
Is scroll through reels of happy faces
People in beautiful places
Love shared between lovers
Breakfasts in bed upon hotel covers
Porcelain skin and perfect bodies
Lavish stays and expensive hobbies.
With every refresh, I sink a bit,
Doomed to watch the world's dark split.
A world my feet cease to touch, yet I so miss.
Doesn't hold air, it doesn't exist
Stop for a moment, take a breath,
Step back from the edge of virtual death.
For the world outside is still and bright—
And beyond the scroll, there's life, there's light.

Hell under heaven

A poem about masking how you feel

I put on my best suit
Only to dress my wound,
Style my hair, I look perfectly pruned.
My god, I look put together
but I know in my heart
No amount of makeup can stop me from falling apart.
I'll walk in, head held high,
Shake hands, strong as I say goodbye.
I'll get home to soon undress,
Stand at the mirror and stare back at this mess,
Get into bed knowing I've tried my best
to not fall to my knees and confess
that I know I hide it well,
But I'm not in heaven – really I'm in hell.

Girl of the trees

A poem about being different

Clubbing and parties were never my scene.
Sure, at the time I acted keen
To look 'cool', to 'fit in'
As I stood there with dread crawling under my skin,
Dreaming of a date with my guitar at home.
I found solace in music and being alone.
I preferred the trees, the birds and the bees,
Running towards the sun against the swift breeze.
Poetry was my party, my notepad and pen.
It's still the best one I've been to, again and again.

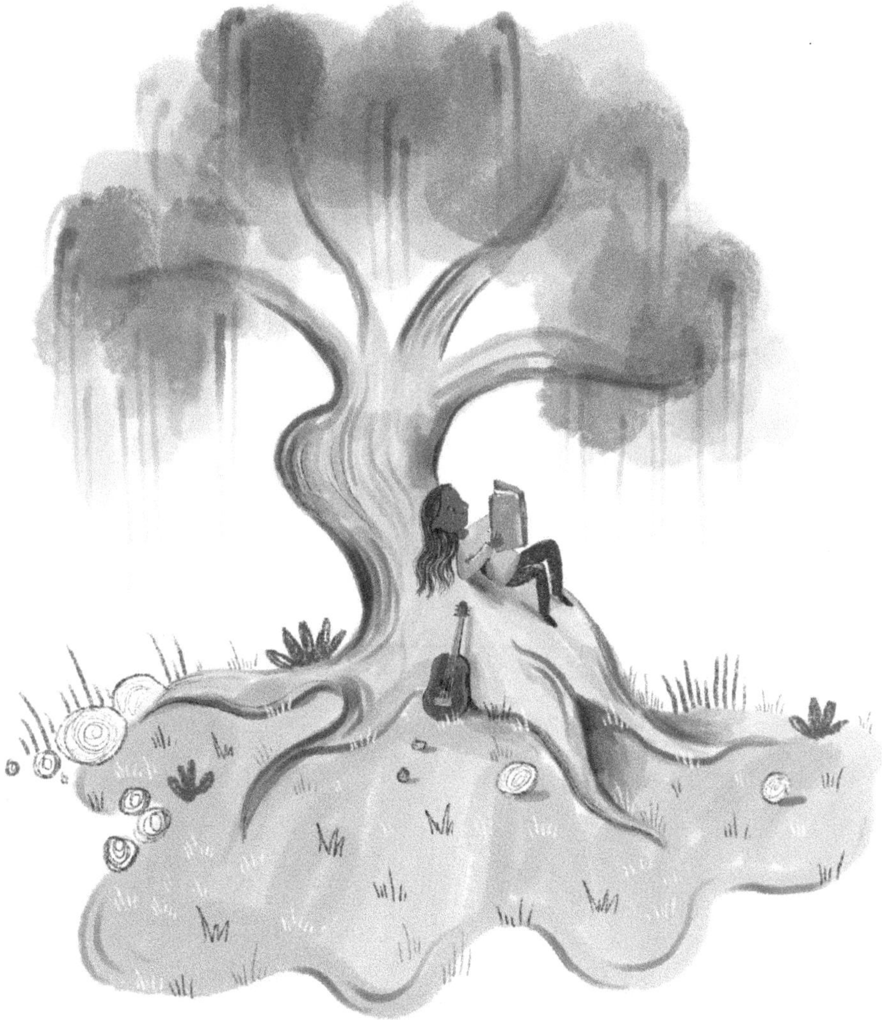

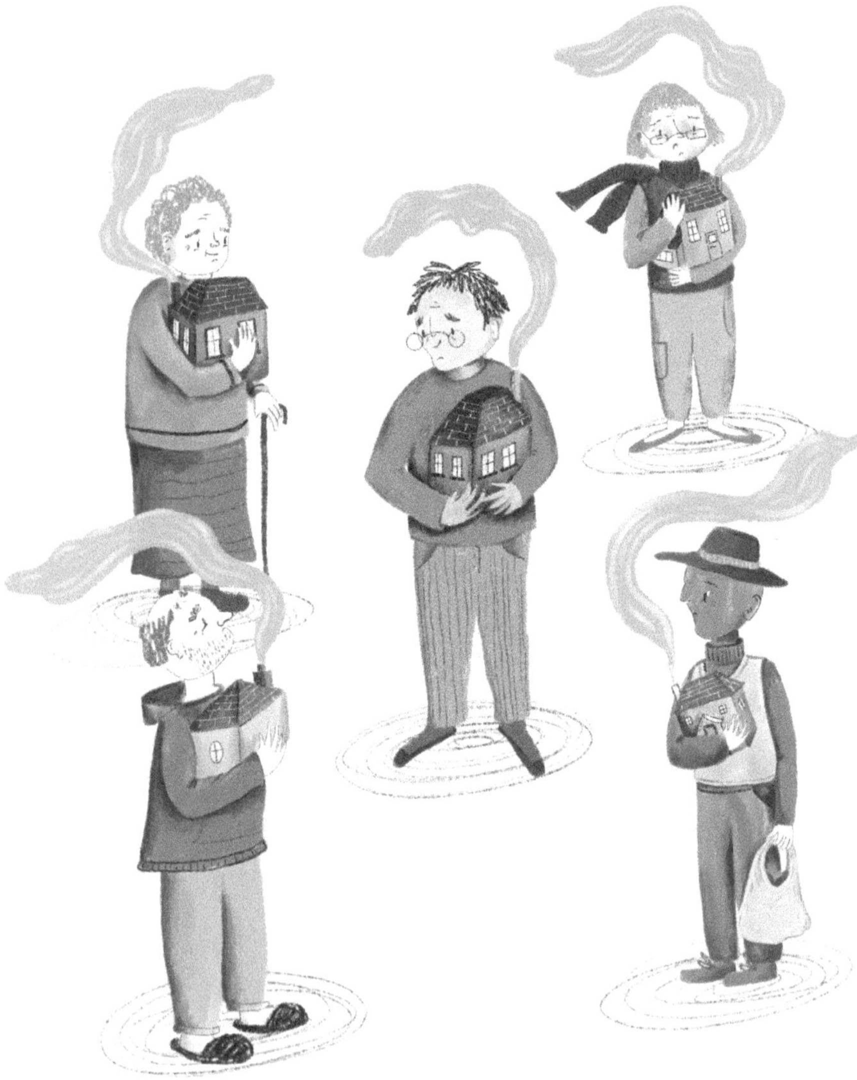

Hollow hours

A poem about loneliness

I sit here having lived a busy life
Cutting my sandwich, I hear the scrape of my knife
as it echoes through the cupboards near
Something I never used to hear
As voices always filled the room
Now it's the frail brushes of my old broom
Or the ripple in my tea
I never thought the sounds of my house would
make me feel so lonely
The only friend I now see is the face on the TV
Or the cashier when I buy milk for my tea
It's funny how life goes so fast until your older years are due
You have all the time in the world but so much less to do
I hope we find each other, if you are reading this poem alone
Even if it's through paper, I'm still sitting here in your home.

Models of diversity

A poem about diversity in the fashion industry

Dedicated to Angel Sinclair, founder of MOD

Beneath me, a platform built for perfection,
Tall, slender, beautiful models with a flawless complexion
To gaze towards and adore somewhere
I never thought would be my floor.
A forbidden place for the soles of my feet
For my face to be beheld as a precious treat
Yet today I've found myself floating through thin air
Showing exquisite garments I have been given to wear
With the intent that I can make them look beautiful.
For society has always told me I would be utterly delusional
To think that I could add any more value to anything I touch
Let alone a silky dress and a velvet diamond clutch.
As this space is home for only a few toes,
For a certain look, for specific clothes,
Not for the ones who are often unspoken.
Unless used as a pull, as an easy token.
I once belonged here, in my youth as they say
Until I found my hair slowly turning grey,
But wouldn't it be so precious to grow old with grace?
To cherish each line which embroiders my face?
Yet I still can't stop thinking, I won't have long left in this space.

A space also home to a brush with one shade.
Not the one I was painted with, as I never made the grade.
Instead of seeing beauty in my roots as the charm of night,
I still can't help but wonder if I would belong more if I was light.
It's funny how we see such magnetism in the diversity of earth
Yet the people who walk among it have been taught since birth
That the skin which lies outside their soul determines their worth
Or the aptitude of their body sets them up for a
bounded existence
In the thought of achievements only being
reachable with assistance.
We all hold scars whether it's in our heart or on our skin,
But isn't that truly a spectacular thing?
Opening the story to the dark places we have been,
and being able to have our courage, to be admired and seen.
If we change our perception of beauty today
My goodness the positive role it will play.
How much more we would have done, if we hadn't felt less,
If we hadn't valued ourselves on fitting into that 'dream dress'.
We've been taken somewhere unreachable, out of grasp.
Even the ones living it cannot make it last.
It is now time to make it real, a space for all.
I don't know about you, but I think that is rather beautiful.
And maybe we don't have to look up and wait for an angel to fall?
Maybe she's down here already, among us all.

I am man

A poem about the unspoken struggles that men experience

It's a weird world out there for me,
As I step out and agonise which version of myself I should be.
Should I be down the gym pumping iron
Instead of at home on my knees crying?
As I lie on my mum's lap,
I cannot help but think I should be down the
pub as the happy chap.
Am I still a man if I love another man?
If I walk down the street holding his hand?
Should I pick up the bill on the first date?
Or is that a patronising, controlling trait?
Can I admit my heart aches for the one I still love?
Can I still be a man and feel all the above?
The answer is yes, yes, I can.
I will and always say, I am a man.

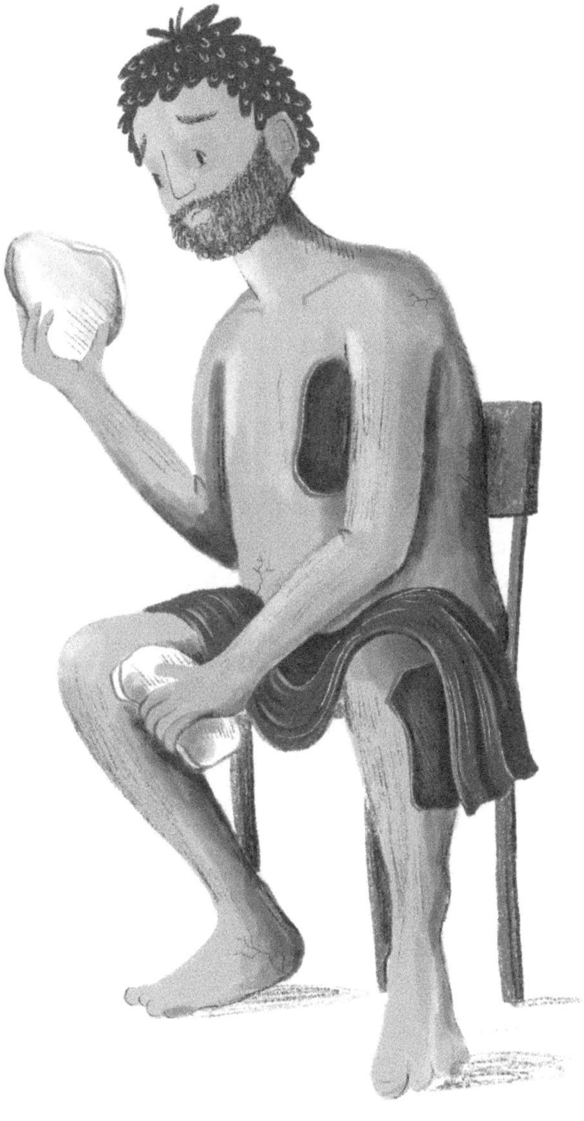

Scroll and hollow

A poem about social media

Once upon a time an innocent idea was created
soon to have the modern world utterly infatuated
A platform for artists to showcase their craft
to share their images draft by draft
We lost ourselves in its heavenly perfection
not taking it as a personal reflection
Magnificent, lined landscapes, objects and people
A place where in our dark days we would recall
Time passed with a turn of events looming
It wasn't just the pictures we found ourselves grooming
Gradually placing ourselves inside the art
Becoming unable to tell each world apart
At that moment we lost sight of everything real
This was when something so beautiful turned evil

My thoughts

Roots

A poem about our environment

At this moment in time, we are living in an extraordinary world,
One which was just a dream that our ancestors once held.
A whole new world has been created through technology –
Instant connections, impeccable images,
a perfect human ideology.
Yet we still go back to the one thing that has always been here,
Nature, the only place we can go without being interfered.
Somewhere craved for and needed yet so effortless and minimal,
A place to go and know that every part is real.
We often sit by the sea in need of time to think in silence,
As it always has a way of bringing us peace and guidance.
Strolling through trees down a muddy
footpath leading to nowhere,
As we catch the rays of sun whilst breathing in the clear air.
Or the calming sound of rain against our windowpanes,
Before the morning rises, we hear the birds sing again.
At these moments we catch ourselves at peace,
in harmony with our roots.
I just hope that, out of both worlds,
the real one we never lose.

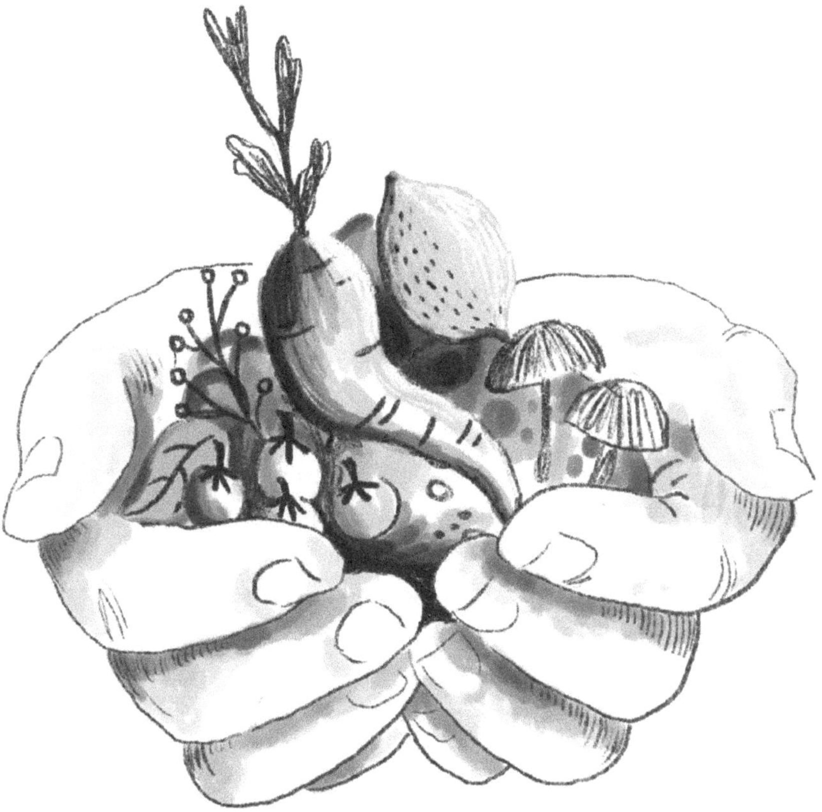

The troll

A poem about cyber bullying

We say 'be kind', but the comments say otherwise.
They take their life, and we act like it's some kind of surprise.
Don't get me wrong, constructive feedback and jokes we need,
But often those which are the loudest are made for us to bleed.
How can we know so little yet can assume so much?
And then we wonder why we have a generation of sad faces,
out of touch.
How can one spit such evil in such bad taste?
As words now can travel without being face to face
Oh, the confidence they must hold behind the screen,
With the quotes they post always saying 'don't be mean',
To hold your head high, that you are a queen.
Yet I know they have people whom they often wish ill.
It doesn't take long for the hatred to spill.
How sad they must be to troll on a stranger and assume
They know the true story, that they can read their room.

Rhyme

A poem about the effects of the modern era

I hope rhyme will always endure the length of time
We hold fast to words so divine
that beauty in language does not fall in vain
I'm frightened the modern era has us conversing all the same
I pray a pen can still hold space upon our table
For soulless gadgets have now become our staple
I know we all need time from what is not true
To be guided back to the simple world we once knew

My thoughts

Poems about the emotional challenges of physical health issues

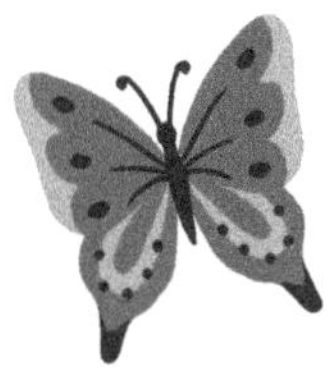

My cage

A poem about Parkinson's disease

Something was out of balance, out of whack
A touch of uneasiness crawling up my back.
It creeps up on you in increments,
A jolt here and there
Sending cracks through your bones which you can't repair.
A body that has held my soul so steadily for so long
I often wonder what I did for it to do me such wrong.
Why did it shrink my world to such a small space?
A much slower, quieter, more limiting place.
I've had many moments of misery with no hope around
As the outlet for my mind has now broken down.
My body has become my cage.
A lifeless performance now fills my stage.
One would have thought silver linings are very few,
but perhaps one has come just when it's due.
I've found; I now take time in my stride,
something I feel that's perhaps on my side.
A much slower life presents
more time with my children and family events.
It's a simpler life, much more enriching.
Less clutter, more appreciative, and more freeing.
I've learnt the art of accepting the wicked and forgiving.
It's a small world for me but thankfully I am still living.

A broken house

A poem about multiple sclerosis

A house where the plumbing stops working,
Jagged edges, furniture keeps jerking,
The yard tilted and is overgrown,
No cable attached to the bedside phone.
Nothing is working as it should, a dismantled home.
I find myself through its walls, for it is now me.
I am no longer a fully functioning body,
Robbed of my only home by cruel MS.
On days I just stay upright at my very best
But it does not have my mind, it does not have all of me.
It will never take my soul as easily as my body.
My stairs can collapse, my roof can cave in,
But I will still stand, even if it's from within.

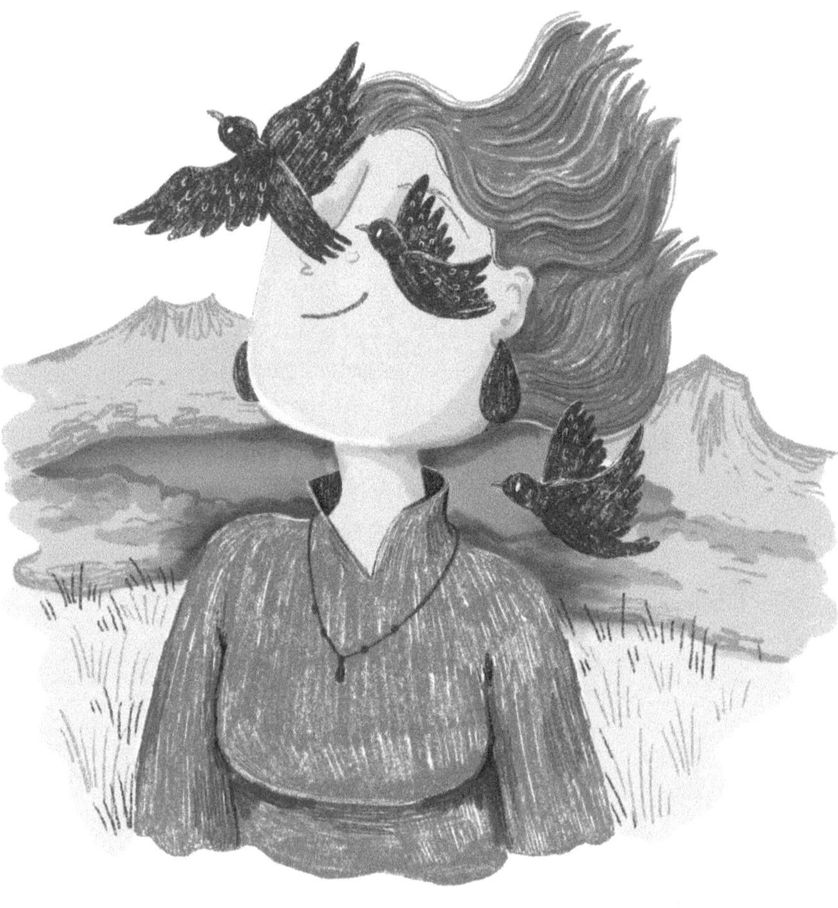

Eyes of the soul

A poem about blindness

I cease to gaze at the morning light.
Still, I can hear birds' tweet to end the night.
The warmth of sun—soft against my skin,
I know this is now where morning begins.
The world, for me, is not in lines
Or green grass to be walked,
But painted in words, by charming ways in which we've talked.
I run through sound, I read by scent,
I feel the smooth and behold the bent.
I'm blessed I would say with a gift that can't be shared,
For I have the magic to only see a human soul bared.
For the shells in which they carry it, you often judge
The soul before it's seen and can all too soon begrudge.
I may not see beauty on the surface of sight,
But I can feel goodness and see mountains in a different light.
Please no pity of difference born
As I live in a world that only my imagination can adorn.

The heat of change

A poem about menopause

In the midst of life's changing tide,
Menopause arrives, a journey to ride.
A phase of transition, a natural shift
Bringing wisdom, grace, a unique gift.
Hormones in flux, emotions run high,
Yet strength emerges as days go by.
Hot flushes, night sweats, a common tale,
Navigating this path, we shall prevail.
Embrace the transformation, the new chapter starts,
Menopause, a metamorphosis of the heart.
With self-care, support, and understanding art,
We embrace this journey, a woman's part.

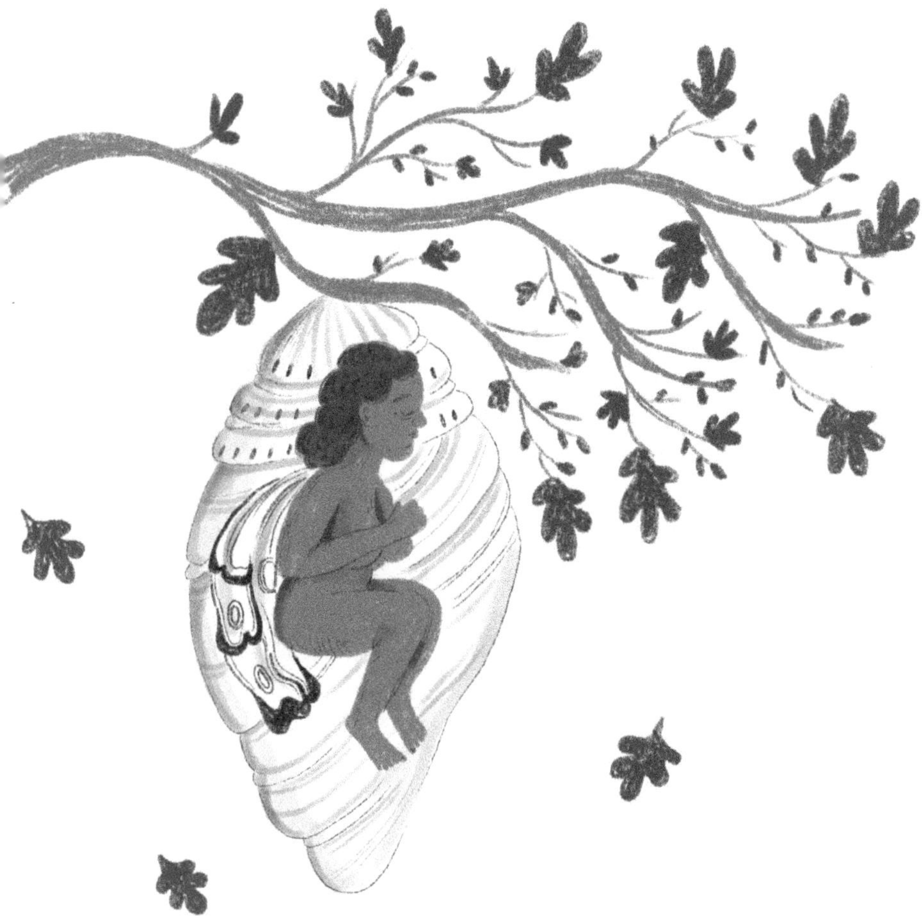

The music I imagine

A poem about deafness

The world is quiet when I wake,
No morning mutters or broken plates,
But silence is not empty air—
It holds a thousand voices there.
My room does not fill with sound,
Just a noise only I have found.
I read your lips and see your eyes.
Through this I hear your cheers and cries.
I feel rhythm through vibrating floors
As guitar strings play and open drawers.
Your hands they gesture your strength and might
For I've learnt to hear much more just through sight.
I've never heard my loved one's cry
But see their pain as they look to the sky
For language lives not only through tone
But through so much more than you've ever known.
So don't mourn the sounds I'll never hear
For it's still a beautiful world for me, don't fear.

The quiet ache

A poem about arthritis

A stiffness, like an iron chain,
holds the body in a battle ground of pain.
A stiffened hand, a limping stride,
The body's strength begins to hide.
Prisoner of my frame I find myself still
For the joy of freedom I can no longer feel.
But though my bones may bend and break,
My mind I will not allow it to take.
Arthritis may wear the body thin,
But the will to live will always keep within,
For strength is not just weaved through bones –
The heart can hold it on its own.

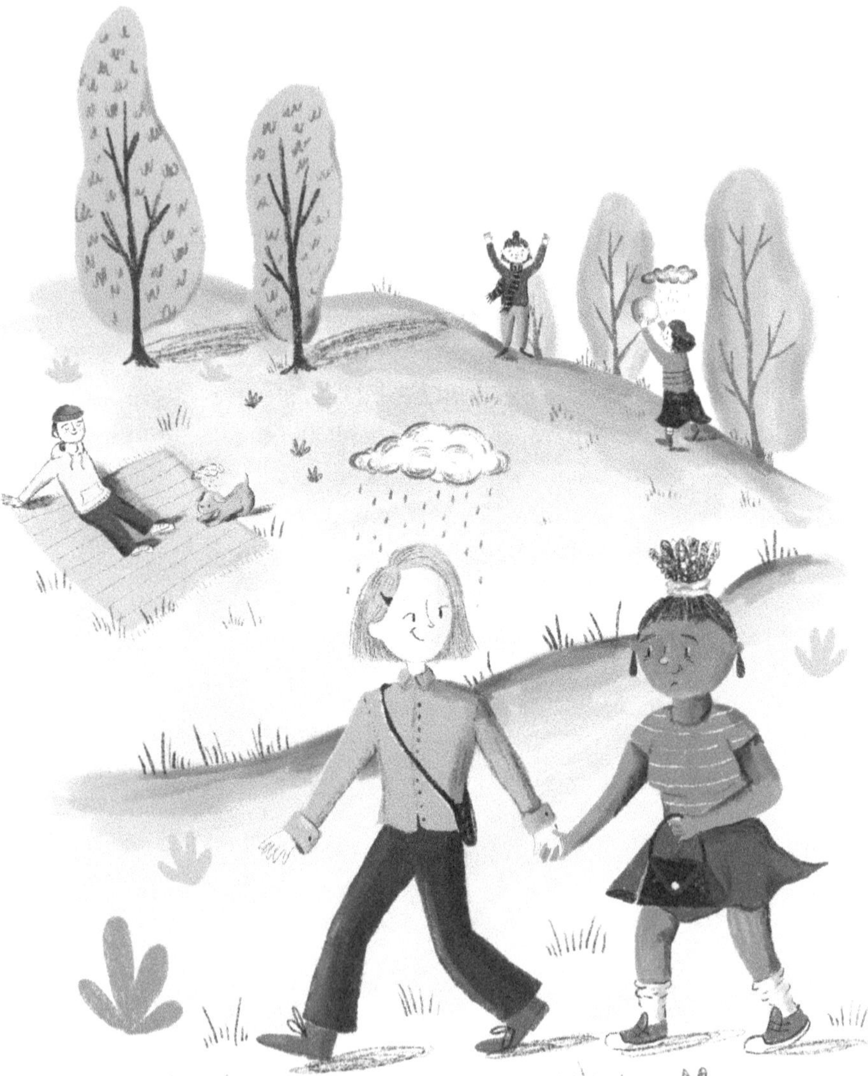

Threads of hope

A poem about cancer

You never think it will be you
that the darkness will set upon.
You always hear about the stories for so long,
Of clouds raining on the wrong people, of the pain,
When cancer crawls in with no shame
But you assume you'll just watch and listen,
As your plans for the future start to glisten.
You take advantage of time being kind,
As small problems take hold of your mind.
Then it arrives, what you never thought would come.
All those minor problems you had are now overtaken by one.
You start to count your days, through thoughts of haze.
At night the sky starts to catch your gaze.
The scent of the lawn smells finer than perfume,
The simple things in life become so in-tune –
The sun, the stars and the moon.
The only good in such bad
Is realising the gifts that you already had.
Keep your strength strong,
Don't let the whispers of your doubt hang around for long
Because your body listens to your mind,
So please, let it be kind.

The weight of waking

A poem about chronic fatigue syndrome

I wake, but not from a restful sleep,
The dawn arrives, yet the morning feels steep.
My bones are heavy, my heart is slow,
Hope rises like a bare-winged crow.
The world expects a brisk walk, a steady mile,
when I can barely forge a willing smile,
But they cease to feel this hidden thief
that steals my motion, robs my belief.
It's not just tired—no, it's more:
a hollow blight pressed into my core.
No sleep, no rest can clear the mist
that surrounds my body as I lift each fist.
Yet I'll never surrender; as days pass by
I'll still rise, even if I can't touch the sky.
For strength is not in speed or stride,
but in the will to stay, abide.
So, if I pause, or seem withdrawn,
know I am fighting from dusk till dawn.

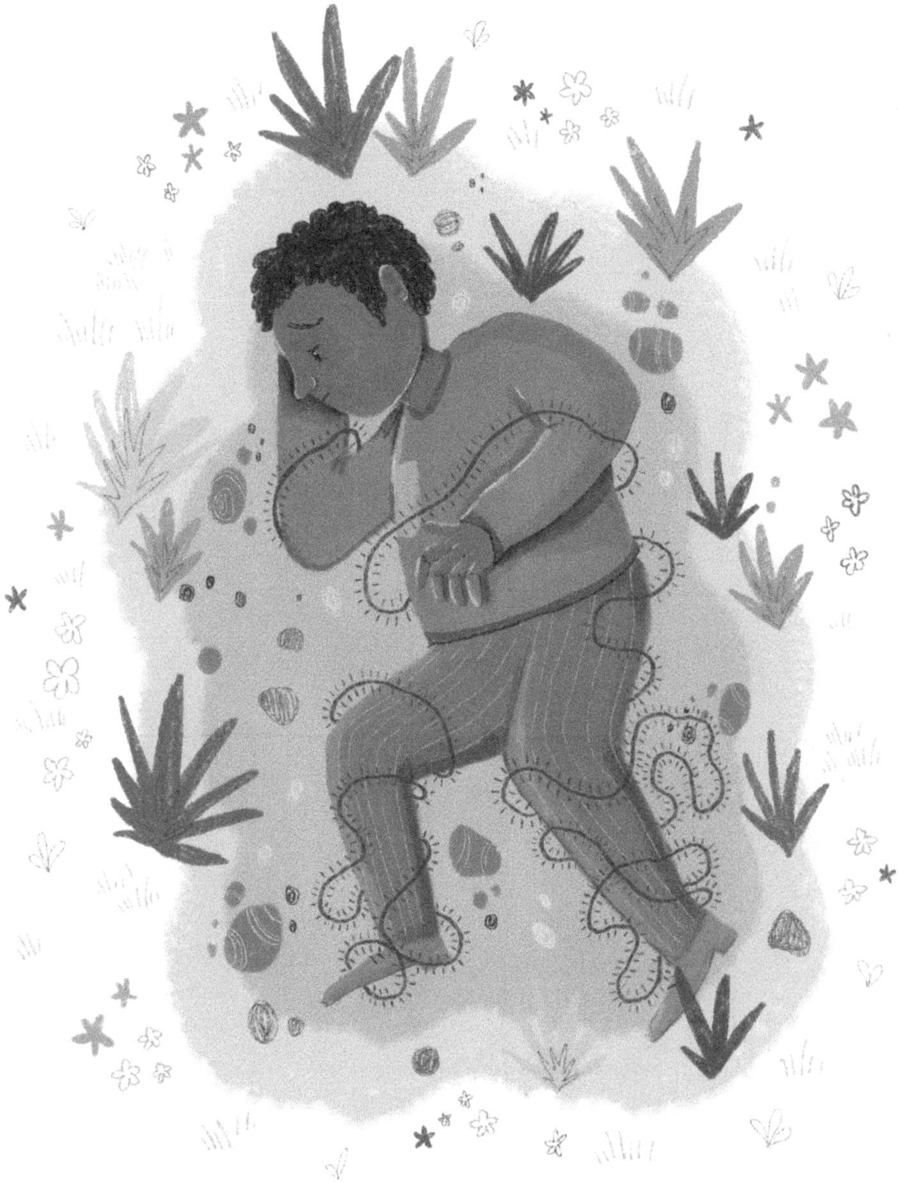

My thoughts

Poems about positivity

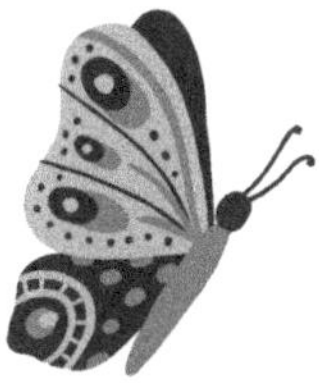

Steady in the storm

From a carer to a sufferer

I can still see it there
In your eyes, your chaotic room, what you wear
Mismatched clothes and unwashed hair
That dark tormented vacant stare
I know it still comes around from time to time
I feel it in your grip as you place your hand in mine
It's okay if the war still lies upon your mind
If the hauntings aren't fully left behind
There's no shame if your battle can still reminisce
For a clean-cut war can often be amiss
I cherish the times when your eyes are clear
That there are now moments you are without fear
But when its evil head does reappear
I promise you I will always be here

Hands that heal

A poem about being kind

Let me help you through.
I see your feet are weary and hurting too
for before me walk your blistered soles.
Like me, life must have taken its toll.
I know not your story, but I know your hope is worn.
I have not walked in your shoes, but I see they are
withered and torn.
Perhaps enough to tell your story so I need not ask.
Kindness, I bet in many times, seemed beyond your grasp.
Although I am empty, I still see your pain,
So put your arm in mine and I'll show you kindness once again.
Let's go slowly, as I said my soles are withered too,
But I'll hold you up, if you'll hold me up
– together we'll make it through.

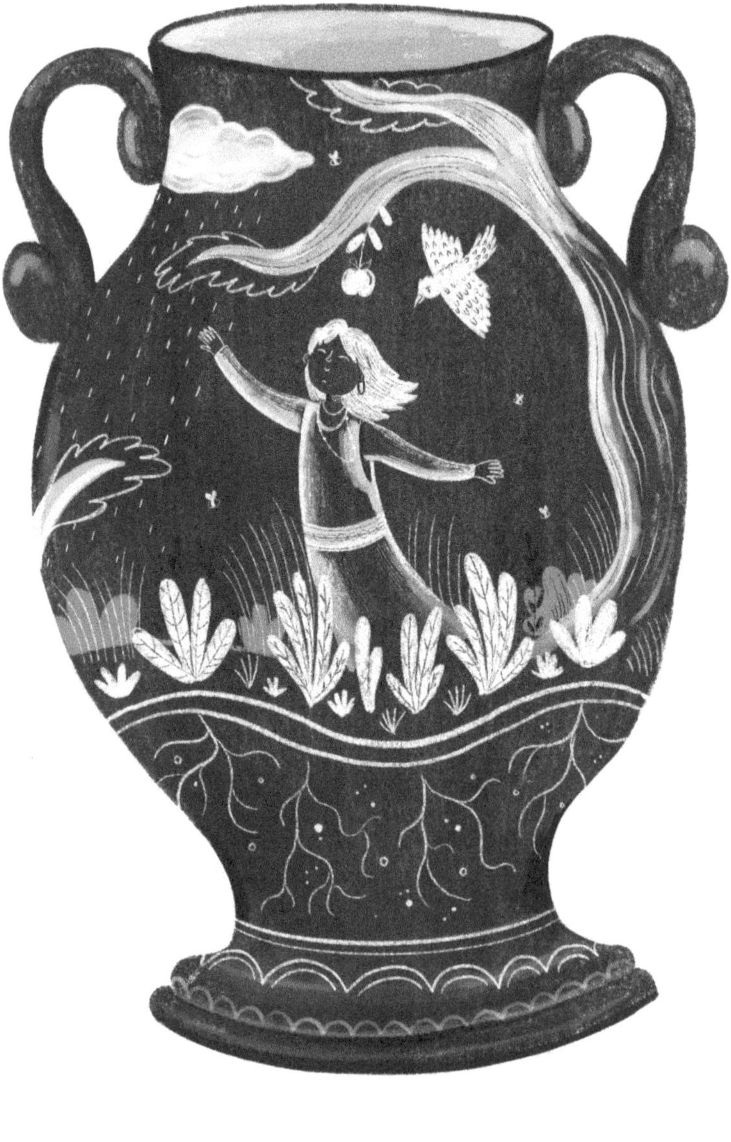

My Gift

A poem about loving your body

I was born here, in this home,
Gifted to my soul so I wouldn't wander alone,
A vessel to see the world, feel the breeze caress my skin
Whilst I taste its fruits as they trickle down my chin.
I can hear the birds, the bees, and the gentle blow
among the trees
As it carries me through the years, through its adversities,
through my tears.
Shouldn't I feel so blessed to have such a miracle carry me?
Yet I can't remember when my vessel became my enemy,
When I started to worry more, about what other people saw,
When the eyes to my soul were no longer my door.
My outside owned every part of my worth
Now isn't that a sad way to walk the earth?
Just remember your body was made to protect your mind
Because your soul is truly the most precious thing in humankind.

I shall not judge

A poem about not judging people

These days I shall not judge anyone
As I myself have bowed down to the devil at times
I mean, I've not committed the act of murderous crimes
But believe me, I've followed the tail of error
Moments out of character inducing immense terror
Times it was out of the question to see
That even I myself couldn't understand me
We all stray from ourselves from time to time
Do things that don't always seem to align
So, who would I be to judge something I don't understand?
I just know the best thing to do is to hold out my hand.

The heart I hold

A poem about self-love

You know, the love we give to ourselves is also free
We seem to give it out to others so eagerly
Yet to ourselves it seems to have such a high price put upon
Used very thinly just in case we are wrong
Because, God forbid, we love ourselves too strong
If only the views we have of our friends
Would allow us to see ourselves through the same lens
What beautiful reflections would fill our mirrors
And kind words would come to our ears
It's only when the years pass us by
Does our self-love seem to become less shy
Maybe one day our love for ourselves will override
The self-doubt that always lies by our side

My lighthouse

From a sufferer to a carer

It's his love that understood
things I thought someone never could.
When darkness seeps through my mind,
And tangled thoughts are all I find,
You reach into the storm I hide,
With an open heart and arms wide.
You never shy at what you see,
Those fraying threads inside of me,
Instead, you hold me within your arms tight,
Speak words that help me get back up and fight.
You don't fix all, you never try
To chase the thunder from the sky,
But still, your voice—a steady breeze—
Brings gentler waters for me to seize.
To walk beside me, not ahead,
To bring me peace, not make me 'better' instead.
Some days I drown in heavy rain,
But you become the guard, my windowpane,
A lighthouse blinking through and through,
My safe return is found in you.
So, when the storms spin through once more,
And hope runs thin as I kneel to the floor,
I know I'll never be alone—
Because with you, I'm always home.

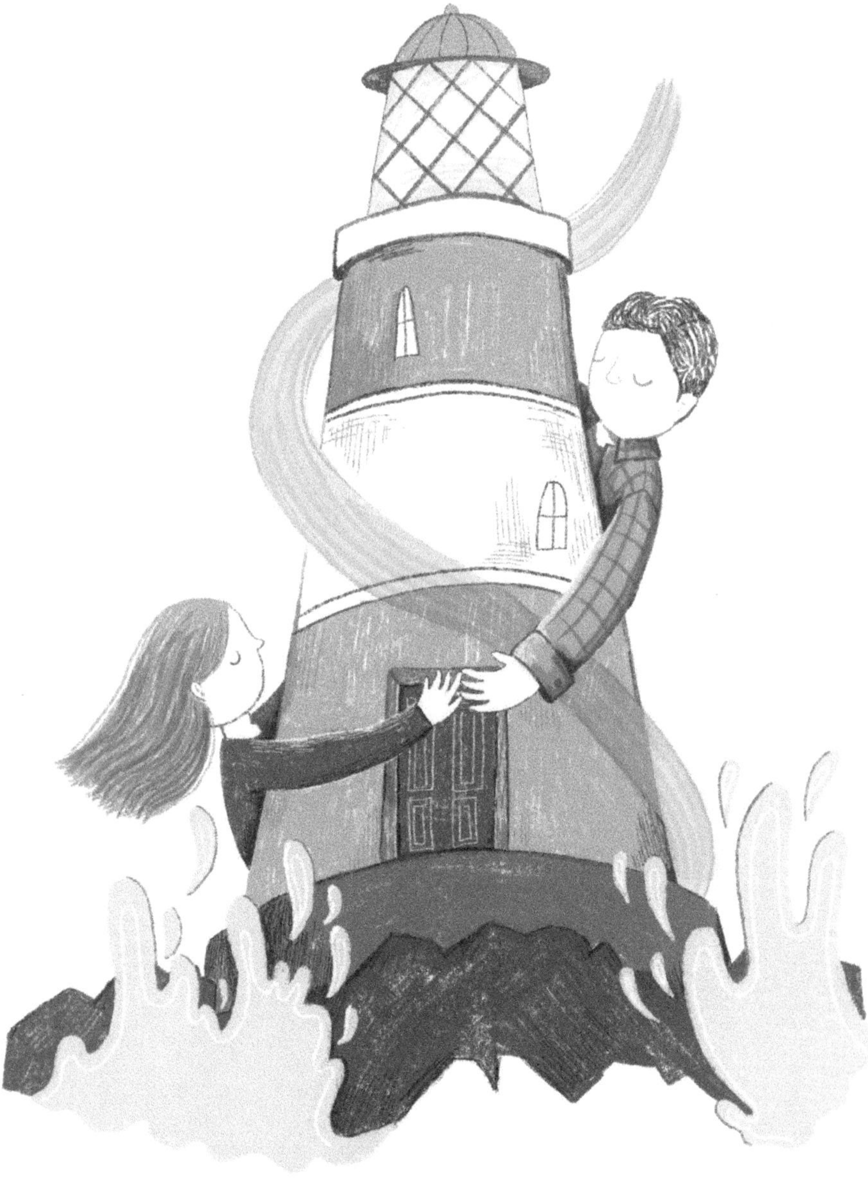

My thoughts

Outside the ring

A poem about self-responsibility

Dedicated to Frank Bruno MBE

As a young kid I was always getting into trouble
I needed something to snap me out of my bubble
I was angry and often felt very alone
Then I put on some gloves and found my home
Boxing became my discipline
Giving me highs when I'd win
Bruise after bruise, when I'd lose
But the motivation became my muse
I was becoming one of the best of my time
Standing on top of the world in all my prime
Gratitude and love ran up and down my spine
In that moment everything seemed to align
But as we all know, nothing lasts forever
Although I seemed to lose everything all together
My marriage came to an end
Money stole my friends
Drugs soon consumed my pain
Unravelling every wire in my brain
Tangling everything that was once sane
I was diagnosed with bipolar and manic depression
Experiencing sudden highs then turns of aggression
None of these changes I could seem to question
Slowly becoming bipolar's perfect possession
I woke up one day to people barging into my home

Coming into my space when I was peacefully alone
Escorting me out as if I'd done something wrong
Every bit of my freedom was immediately gone
As for my dignity, that didn't take long
The way they treated me inside as a patient
It was like I was some ugly creature found in a basement
I was worthless, just a hindrance to their day
Just a task they had to get out of the way
And the quicker it was done the shorter I'd stay
Not once did they talk about the thoughts in my head
It was easier for them to leave me sedated in my bed
It was like they were afraid of what they couldn't see
The voices in my head were what was wrong with me
which made it impossible for them to set me free
It was easier to turn me into a silent zombie
Unable to speak out on what was happening to me
They treated me like a lab rabbit
Feeding me tablet after tablet
which knocked me for six after I'd had it
Injection after injection, drug after drug
Just brushing all my demons under a rug
I was a prisoner within my own head
My thoughts chaining me to my bed
One moment away from being brain dead
I went back to the one thing that had saved me before
The only thing that always made me really want more
Something that has built me up from my core
Boxing, exercise and the gym
Something that has always released my demons from within
I started to eat right
Sleep well at night
Look after my body and mind
My medicine was all of these elements combined

As well as the fighter within my soul
Pulling me out of this malicious black hole
I have fought some of the strongest battles in the ring
But I never thought I would have to challenge one from within
One that exceeded every fight I'd had before
An endless unforgiving inside war
Mental illness can hold anyone in captivity
But I also know everyone holds their own key
Somewhere there is always hope of setting yourself free
We must find a solution that can cure the problem,
not just hide it
We need to listen to the voice inside it
And then we will find a route to a cure
We have to speak out to be able to win this tortuous war

Where the stars whisper hope

A poem about hope

It's the stars that tell us who we are
Because they have always watched us, from afar
They see us in our most unshielded hours away from the day
The ones where we may cry, clench our fists or pray
There's something about the dark, as we sit in the depths of night
The stars will come out, to remind us there's still light
A beautiful moment in time as we gaze up at the sky
As the questions we ask them, unlike humans, they will never lie.

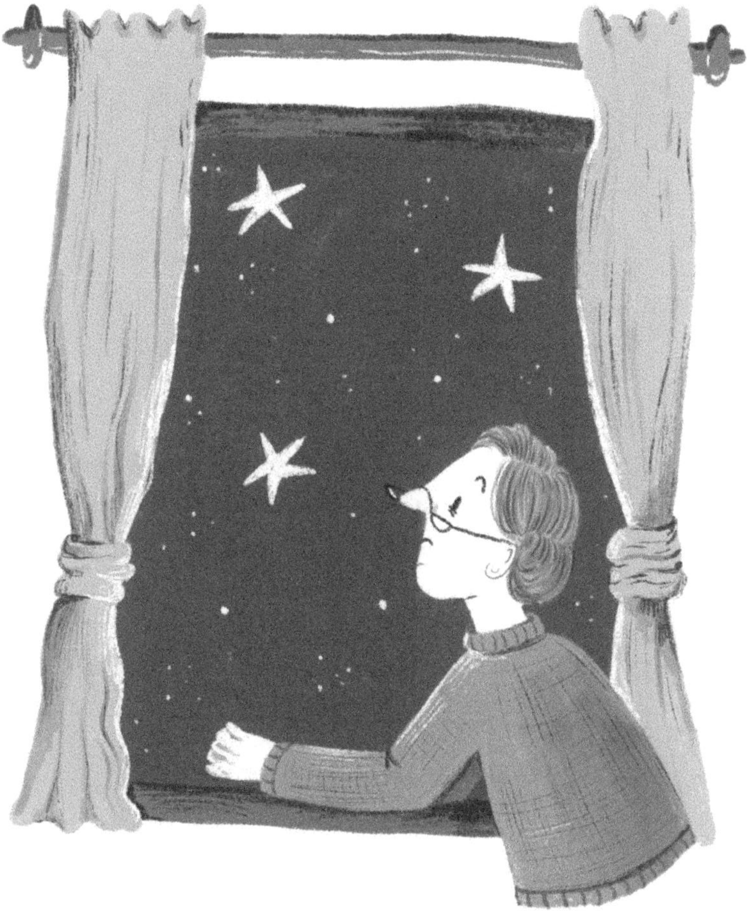

We all bleed the same

A poem about communities coming together

We may look different as our skin can first show,
We may come from afar, from across the globe,
We may talk unalike as we first speak,
Seem like strangers upon our first meet,
But one thing we do share is the same mother beneath our feet.
She made us to be diverse so we could excite the earth,
But none of our differences should ever determine our worth.
If one could see beauty in their roots as the charm of night,
Not wonder if they would belong more if they were light.
For Mother Nature never intended for the human
race to be divided
For the hands of power to be one sided
Or for one's value to be weighed upon the pigment in one's skin
But only to be judged by the attributes within.
As voiced by the commendable Martin Luther King
We are made by our soul, the courage of our mind,
In our ability to be brave, generous, and kind.
We all spill tears through our eyes, love and feel pain.
We are all one, we all bleed the same.

Malcolm

A poem about someone's belief in you

There's a light that shines, not from the skies
But from a soul who came by surprise
Stood across the road was a kind-looking man
He smiled hello with a suitcase in hand
Strangers at first so it seemed
Till he spilled his suitcase full of dreams
Dreams which came with no cost
Just empowerment and belief which I had lost
For every artist, dreamer, friend,
There is one soul who helps them mend.
And all the stars that burn anew
Where faith was restored by angels like you

Resources and support

ANDY'S MAN CLUB

Email: Info@andysmanclub.co.uk
Instagram: @andysmanclubuk   https://andysmanclub.co.uk/

Andy's Man Club is a suicide prevention charity, offering free-to-attend peer-to-peer support groups across the United Kingdom and online. Aiming to end the stigma surrounding men's mental health and help men through the power of conversation.

ALZHEIMER'S SOCIETY

Dementia support: 0300 222 11 22
Instagram: alzheimerssoc   https://www.alzheimers.org.uk/

Alzheimer's Society is the UK's leading dementia charity. They campaign for change, fund research to find a cure and support people living with dementia today.

CANCER RESEARCH UK

Email: supporter.services@cancer.org.uk
Telephone: 0300 123 1022 Instagram: @cr_uk
https://www.cancerresearchuk.org/

Cancer research UK is the world's leading independent charity dedicated to saving lives through research. Its website is a source of authoritative, up-to-date information about cancer and its treatment.

CHATTY CAFÉ SCHEME

Email: Abi@thechattycafescheme.co.uk
Instagram: @thechattycafe   https://thechattycafescheme.co.uk/

The Chatty Café Scheme is the UK's leading non-profit organisation tackling loneliness. It offers three services, all designed to reduce loneliness and/or social isolation:

1. Face-to-face meet ups
2. Online Chatty sessions
3. Telephone friendship service

CRUSE BEREAVEMENT CARE

Helpline: 0808 808 1677(see website for opening hours)
Instagram: @crusesupport   https://www.cruse.org.uk/

Cruse helps people through one of the most painful times in life – with bereavement support, information and campaigning.

DEMENTIA UK

Helpline: 0800 888 6678 or
helpline@dementiauk.org   dementiauk.org

Dementia UK is the specialist nursing charity that provides support for the whole family. Its nurses are known as Admiral Nurses and provide free life-changing support and advice to anyone affected by dementia.

FIRST STEPS ED

Email: info@firststepsed.co.uk

Instagram: @firststepsed https://firststepsed.co.uk/

A charity supporting children, young people, adults, and their families affected by eating difficulties and disorders.

FRANK BRUNO FOUNDATION

Email: info@thefrankbrunofoundation.co.uk

Instagram: @frankbrunofoundation

https://www.thefrankbrunofoundation.co.uk/

The Frank Bruno Foundation exists to provide support and encouragement and the motivation to succeed for those currently facing or recovering from mental ill-health issues. The Foundation aims to achieve this by providing opportunities to participate in a well-being and non-contact boxing program, supported by a needs-led wrap-around service. The Foundation directly supports participants in building self-esteem, confidence, resilience and discipline and in applying such skills to their daily lives. It campaigns to raise public awareness of mental ill-health and how this can affect anyone at any time and to knock out the stigma surrounding this using its social media platforms and its charity ambassadors to encourage anyone facing mental ill-health to talk openly and not to feel discriminated against.

HOARDING DISORDERS UK

Email: Info@hoardingdisorders.org
Instagram: @Hoardingdisordersuk
https://hoardingdisordersuk.org/

Specialist advice for people affected by hoarding behaviours, chronic disorganisation and extreme clutter.

MACMILLAN CANCER SUPPORT

Telephone: 0808 808 00 00 – 7 days a week,
8 am-8 pm, calls are free in the UK
Instagram: @macmillancancer
https://www.macmillan.org.uk/

Macmillan Cancer Support is one of the largest British charites. It provides specialist health care, information and financial support to people affected by cancer It also looks at the social, emotional and practical impact cancer can have, and campaigns for better cancer care. Its goal is to reach and improve the lives of everyone affected by cancer in the UK.

MARMALADE TRUST

Email: info@marmaladetrust.org
Instagram: @marmalade_trust
https://www.marmaladetrust.org/

The Marmalade Trust is an award-winning charity dedicated to raising awareness of loneliness and empowering people to make connections.

NATIONAL AUTISTIC SOCIETY

Telephone: 0207 833 2299
Instagram: @nationalautisticsociety
https://www.autism.org.uk/

The National Autistic Society is the UK's leading charity for autistic people and their families. Since 1962, it has been providing support, guidance and advice. It works to transform lives and change attitudes to help create a society that works for autistic people.

RNIB (ROYAL NATIONAL INSTITUTE OF BLIND PEOPLE)

Contact: https://www.rnib.org.uk/about-us/contact-us/
Instagram: @rnib https://www.rnib.org.uk/

RNIB, is the UK's leading sight loss charity. It offers practical and emotional support to blind and partially-sighted people, their families and carers. It raises awareness of the experiences of blind and partially-sighted people and campaign for change to make society more accessible for all.

MODELS OF DIVERSITY

Contact: https://modelsofdiversity.org/
Instagram: @modelsofdiversity
Email: info@modelsofdiversity.org

Campaigning for representation in the media, beauty and fashion industry.

RNID (ROYAL NATIONAL INSTITUTE FOR DEAF PEOPLE)

Telephone: 0808 808 0123 Email: contact@rnid.org.uk.
Instagram: rnid_uk https://rnid.org.uk/

RNID is the UK's national charity supporting more than 18 million people in the UK who are deaf, have hearing loss or tinnitus.

SAMARITANS

Telephone: 116 123 Email: admin@samaritans.org
Instagram: @samaritancharity https://www.samaritans.org/

The Samaritans offer a safe place for you to talk anytime about anything that is worrying you. They are available round the clock, 24 hours a day, 365 days a year and it is free to call within the UK.

SANE

Email: support@sane.org.uk
General enquiries: 0203 805 1790 (office hours)
Email: info@sane.org.uk Instagram: @charitysane
https://www.sane.org.uk/
Helpline: 0300 304 7000 – 4 pm-10 pm, 365 days a year
Call-back number: 0300 124 7900 (leave your first name and phone number; they will call you back)

SANE is a leading UK mental health charity improving quality of life for anyone affected by mental illness.

Acknowledgments

I would like to say a big thank you to my wonderful mum and dad, for always believing that recovery is possible and for giving me the freedom to follow my dreams.

Charlotte, my loyal and loving twin sister, the dedication to this book says everything I need to say.

Thank you too to my gorgeous niece and nephew, Georgia and Reggie, who have brought endless light and laughter into our family.

Thank you to Mark for stepping up when I needed you the most and for being you.

Thank you Callum for being the brother I never had.

Also to my grandparents, especially my grandma who is my best friend from another era.

Thank you to all my friends, especially my best friend Zoe, Alice and Lillie, my creative partner.

Over the years I have been incredibly blessed to have been supported by so many wonderful people from all walks of life; for this I am and will always be extremely grateful.

Last but by no means least, thank you to Georgina Bentliff (Hammersmith Health Books) for being supportive, open-minded and a pleasure to work with.

Index

addiction, 40
ADHD, 55
ageing, 37
anorexia nervosa, 44
arthritis, 89
anxiety, 60
bipolar, 41
blindness, 85
bulimia, 59
cancer, 91
carer-sufferer relationship, 96, 102
chronic fatigue syndrome, 92
community, 110
cyber bullying, 78
deafness, 88
dementia, 53
diversity, 70
eating disorders, 32, 44, 50, 59
environment, 76
father, 16
fitting in, 66
gender dysphoria, 45
grandmother, 19
grief, 36
heartbreak, 31
hoarding disorder, 47
hope, 109
kindness, 97
loneliness, 69
masking feelings, 65
medication, 54
menopause, 86
men's mental health challenges, 72
mental illness, general, 42, 56
modern life challenges, 79
mother, 20
multiple sclerosis, 83
OCD, 58
over-thinking, 28
pets, 22
Parkinson's disease, 82
PTSD, 48
self-love, 99, 101
Social media, dark side of, 64, 74
twins, 2, 15

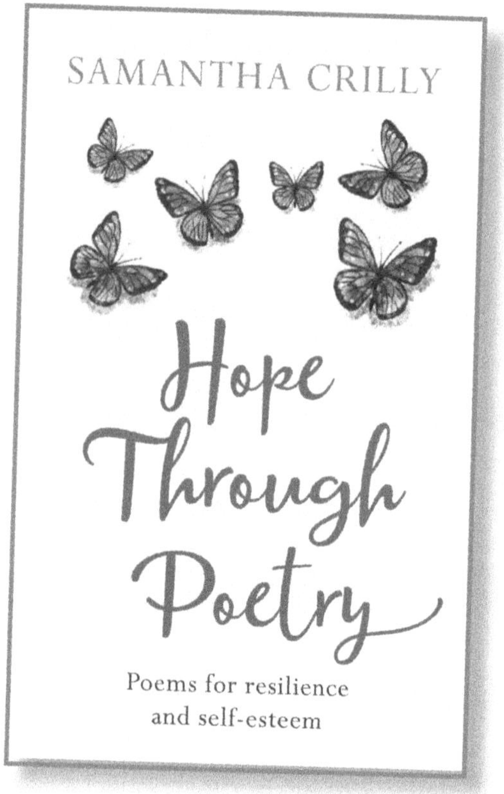

Samantha's first collection of poems sprang from her own experience of, and recovery from, an eating disorder and OCD. Aimed at encouraging resilience and self-esteem in the face of life's many challenges, her poetry has brought comfort and strength to many, both on the page and in performance.

Instagram @samantha_jade_crilly
Tik Tok @samanthacrilly